Brave Beautiful Birth

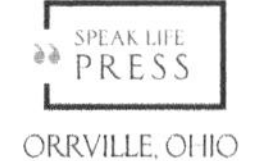

ORRVILLE, OHIO

Brave Beautiful Birth: Trusting God Through VBAC

Jaimie M. Schrock

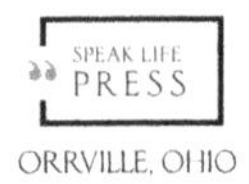

This book is not intended to be used as medical advice. Please consult your healthcare provider to address your specific health needs.

Publishing and Design Services: MelindaMartin.me

Author Photo: SummerKellogg.com

ISBN: 978-1-7322536-0-5 (print)

Brave Beautiful Birth

TRUSTING GOD THROUGH VBAC

JAIMIE M. SCHROCK

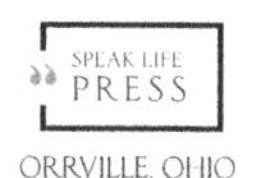

ORRVILLE, OHIO

Dedication

I dedicate my story to my God. He is a good Father and through this has taught me to speak His Word and trust His heart.

I dedicate this book to my loving, encouraging husband who has seen me struggle and wrestle my thoughts and fears during my fourth pregnancy. Thank you for pointing my eyes back to the One true God. You have been a solid rock and encourager to me. Thank you for helping me in every way. I love you.

I dedicate this book to my children. You have taught me more than you will ever know. I love you deeper than deep. You are my crown.

To my sister and best friend, Lyndsey, who is always there for me. I love you. I'm so thankful for you. Thank you for listening to my endless thoughts, concerns, and questions I just need to get out. Our solid, steady friendship means the world to me.

To my family and friends, new and old. Without you, I couldn't have this story. Your words, whether few and seldom or often and many, have helped me in ways you will never know. Thank you.

To my doula, chiropractor, and doctor, I thank you. I know you were hand chosen for this season in my life. Thank you for the many ways you made my story possible. My heart is very thankful for you.

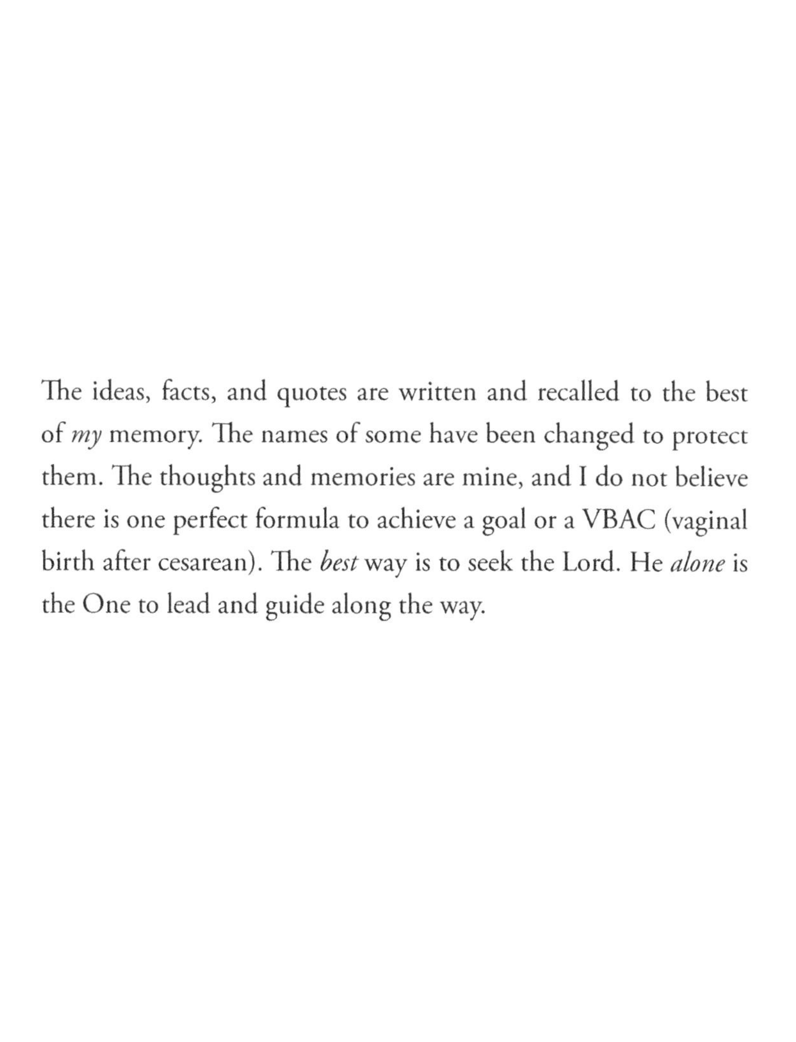

The ideas, facts, and quotes are written and recalled to the best of *my* memory. The names of some have been changed to protect them. The thoughts and memories are mine, and I do not believe there is one perfect formula to achieve a goal or a VBAC (vaginal birth after cesarean). The *best* way is to seek the Lord. He *alone* is the One to lead and guide along the way.

Contents

Preface

I write this to honor my God. To tell His story, His greatness, His power. To give Him glory for the great works He has done, to honor Him, and to bring praise to His name. I write this for Him.

I write this for me. I write this to process all that has happened, this great turning point in my life. To put it on paper has helped me better grasp the beautiful ways that the Lord God worked in my life. This has been good for my soul to remember what He has done, and it has allowed my faith to grow so that I will continue to trust Him in the future.

I write this to you, dear mother, who longs and wants a VBAC desperately. You and I know this path. We know the millions of thoughts and fears that run through our minds, those thoughts that keep us awake at night. I write to you, dear one, who struggles for the most important people in your life to understand you, to understand this deep, intense desire that many say you are crazy for feeling. I write this for you.

I write this for you, dear reader, who is longing to trust Him in a deeper way than you have before in your life. I write this to encourage you to trust Him even more. He speaks. He moves. He loves you, and He can be trusted. I write this to encourage you to throw your fears aside and run to Him. Run to the One who can take those fears and smash them and expose His truth. He is the great Shepherd who comforts us. I pray you will fear no evil, for He is with you. His rod and His staff comfort you. May you know His love, His power, and His faithfulness more after reading what He has done for me.

Oh give thanks to the Lord,
call upon His name;

Make known His deeds among the peoples.
Sing to Him, sing praises to Him;
Speak of all His wonders.
Glory in His holy name;
Let the heart of those who
seek the Lord be glad.
Seek the Lord and His strength;
Seek His face continually.
Remember His wonderful deeds
which He has done...

—I Chronicles 16:8-12

Acknowledgements

Thank you to my editor, Sarah Jones. You are so talented and I respect you so much, in so many ways. Thank you for helping me and being so positive throughout the process.

Thank you to Mary L. Cooper, community midwife, and Amber Piller, Professional Birth Doula, for your help. I appreciate you both so very much.

Thank you to Jessica Smartt, for giving me the opportunity to share on the *Smartter Each Day* blog. It has opened great doors for me and has been a gift. Thank you.

One

"The doctor will be here shortly," the nurse says to me. "He's running behind..."

I lie there in the bed they wheeled me in, shivering — partly because of the cold, hospital air, and partly because of the fear within me. I lie there, a few feet away from being inside the operating room. Waiting. Watching the nurses lay out sharp, shiny tools, and many towels.

"I can't do this," I say to my husband. "I can't do this, I'm scared. I want to get out of here." I look at him from under the shower cap-looking hat upon my head. I look into his eyes, trying to speak the words I don't even know how to say — an attempt to explain the anxiety that causes my heart to beat faster and my skin to sweat.

He smiles at me while leaning on the bed railing. "We have to do this. We have no other options."

It was a rainy, chilly fall day. We left our home and our two children with my dad early in the morning to be at the hospital on schedule so I could be prepped for surgery. We had all posed for a quick picture before Ben and I, bags packed, left for the hospital.

They were so cute. So little. Two blonde boys I couldn't love any more than I already did. We kissed them and hugged them, hugged my dad, and assured them we would see them soon.

"I'm so tired … am I supposed to be this tired?" I ask the assistant, standing on the other side of my bed. "Did they give me something to make me feel tired?" He shakes his head *no* to me as we wait in front of the operating room, doors open.

No. I am so tired because I was awake all night praying I would go into labor instead of having to show up on this day for my scheduled cesarean section. I was having a great pregnancy. I felt great. With only 20 pounds gained and still feeling active and strong, I felt like neither I nor my baby was ready for this to be her birthday.

From my first baby, born at 36 weeks, I knew every day counted. Every day that baby stays inside the precious warm womb the healthier she is, the easier the breastfeeding, and the better able her body is to regulate her temperature. I wanted and wished SHE could pick her birthday. But we sat there, scheduled around the doctor and the hospital. And because doctors are busy helping many people, they can often be late — which was the case this day.

This was the longest I had ever been pregnant. I wondered what the beginning of labor would look like had I had the opportunity to experience it. Would my water have broken? Would I have had contractions start like my second pregnancy? I felt robbed. This was supposed to be about me. This was *my* life. I wasn't sick. I had no health issues. Yet, I wasn't in control, and there I was, having a baby in a way in which I was not comfortable. I wanted to cry. But would anyone understand? Even come to my aid? I felt helpless.

Lying there, waiting and watching the nurses prep, anxiety set in — making its way from my mind to my body — an all-over panic. I wanted to run — I felt the genuine urge to flee. Why does it have to be this way? I had hoped to feel joy in this moment, but the thought of surgery instead had taken my mind away from the beautiful gift I was about to receive.

"He will be here any minute," she says to us again as she walks by. The nurse was doing her everyday job. This was nothing special to her. But today was to be special for *me*. It was the day *my* baby would be born — an event that would never happen again. This would be a sacred day in our lives, even if it wasn't the way I had pictured.

You never forget birth — the moment that baby comes into the world, leaving her mother's body to breathe on her own. Her body begins to work in a new way as it adapts to life outside. It is so special, so amazing — a holy experience, as life and breath come from God alone. He knit each of us together. He orchestrates new life and all the possibilities it holds for the future.

An older man dressed in scrubs and carrying a clipboard approaches my bedside as I lie there, trying to calm down, telling myself I should be joyful rather than afraid.

"Here. You can go ahead and sign here." He points to the line with the pen, his hands obviously shaking. "This just explains the risks of anesthesia and so forth." He makes a joke which I find no humor in. I have no laughter, or even focus, in me. My mind is aware of and processing my surroundings, but my appetite is not for humor.

I sign — I consent to the risks. I think there might be a list of them, but I'm not really able to focus and read them. And this man ... how old is he? His unsteady hands don't quiet the nerves within me, as he will be the one to administer the needle in my spine. Wonderful. *Please* get it in the right place, I think to myself. *Please.*

And then I hear his voice. My doctor has arrived. He is already in his scrubs. He moves quickly, but not in a rushed way since I'm not in labor and there is no emergency.

"OK," says Eric the assistant. He starts to push my bed in through the doors of the operating room. "We can take you in now."

Well, this is it. No turning back.

I don't say anything to Ben, who is guided into an attached room with a large window that almost covers the wall. Lying flat on my back, I hear the doctor talking and getting ready. I see him out of the corner of my eye, and he appears to be looking over paperwork. I know that soon the surgery will start. For all of them, this is so routine. But this is my life. And I wish I wasn't doing it this way.

I am instructed to hunch over so that the anesthesiologist has the best chance at getting the right spot next to my spine. And he does. The needle goes in effortlessly and easily.

The doctor and nurses are still moving about. One of them comes to insert a catheter, which, thankfully, I could not feel.

Still, so nervous, I lie there, no peace within me. This isn't the way I want it to be, but do I have a choice? This is major surgery, my third cesarean, and I know the procedure well.

I feel thankful for my precious baby — our first girl. My heart is in love with her already. I want to be excited with joy and anticipation.

"Can you feel this?" Roger the anesthesiologist asks.

"No."

He continues to check different places, asking again what I can feel. All is well — I am numb from my chest down and one step closer to seeing my baby. With Ben now back by my side, the doctor starts. I of course don't feel much of anything, but I lie there, looking at the green drape hanging in front of me, and listen. Dr. Hale and Eric the assistant start chatting about meaningless topics while I await the birth of my daughter.

"Sit down," Roger says to Ben, harshly. "You can't be standing there. You need to sit down."

He sounds mean — to the point that somehow I felt like the one in trouble. Ben sits down on the chair next to me and stops peering over the green drape serving as a wall between my eyes and where my baby will emerge. I almost feel scolded, shameful even, though I know I shouldn't. I am a rule follower. I don't like to upset people. So when someone in authority, like an anesthesiologist, tells you to sit down, in my mind you better sit down.

But can I blame my husband for standing? Who doesn't want to witness the birth of his child and catch the first glimpse? Isn't that our right as parents?

Looking back and forth between the curtain and the ceiling,

with a curved white instrument softly blowing oxygen in my face, I wait in anticipation as I feel the all-too-familiar tugging on my stomach. Pressure. More pressure. Pulling. The pulling is hard enough that my whole body moves slightly. I feel the sensation of a large weight leaving my midsection as she is pulled from inside me, making her grand entrance into bright lights and a cold room.

The baby is out. No longer a part of my physical body. The placenta would be taken out and the cord cut — without our eyes having seen any of it.

"She's here. A little girl," announces the doctor. I could tell he was smiling through his words. He was happy for us.

"Is everything OK?"

"Yes, we will just get you all stitched up, and you will be good."

"Please go with the baby," I tell Ben as she is taken from the room to get her vitals checked, and to be cleaned and weighed. Roger is still by my head, monitoring my heartbeat, blood pressure, and other stats.

My sweet baby is here, and I am excited to leave the operating room and just be with her. The doctor and his assistant finish taking care of me while I listen to the cries of my newborn. After some time, the nurse, Ben, and baby return to my side. Little one is wrapped in the standard white hospital blanket with teal and pink lines, a pink hat upon her head. Her face touches mine as the nurse brings her close. Her long fingers moving back and forth, she almost seems to be cooing. I talk to her and say hello, telling her I love her, unable to hold her in my arms. She is wide-eyed and alert, safe and healthy. And for that I am thankful.

Who is this little person? Who will she become? We didn't even know her name yet, but I was so thrilled and excited to have another baby. So blessed — what a joy to have the privilege of being entrusted with another precious life.

She and Ben then disappear, and the doctor leans over as he is finished and getting ready to leave. "All is well. You have very little scar tissue."

"So, I can have more children?" I ask with my head tilted back, in order to fully see his face, which was almost behind me now.

"Yes, you are a great candidate and can have many more c-sections. Everything looks great. In fact, you could have eight more c-sections if you wanted to," he says with a smile.

I almost feel proud that I have no scar tissue, as if I had any part in it.

"Thank you," I tell him as he leaves the room. "Thank you for everything." I was so glad it was over.

Relief comes over me. I always wanted a big family, but, at the same time, I'm not sure I could do this again. Although thankful with the outcome thus far, the anxiety from this birth has been almost more than I could handle. Was it because I didn't have any hormones flowing through my body to signal I was truly ready to have this baby? Or was it all in my mind?

After being transferred off the operating table and into a bed, I am wheeled into my recovery room with baby in the plastic bassinet — Ben following right next to me. Upon my entrance, I am immediately greeted by my sweet friend, who brought me a favorite Starbucks coffee, my sister, mother, and extended family. Feeling half there, I nurse my baby and am checked on by the anesthesiologist, who again makes some bad jokes I find nowhere near funny. I am thankful to hold my precious baby in my arms, but I feel out of it — not like myself.

Soon, my father and children arrive ready to meet and hold her. The pictures we have now are treasures to me, as I don't remember much of what happened. The Demerol I was given made me feel sleepy, sweaty, and sick to my stomach. *Please don't let me throw up*, I remember thinking. I drifted off to sleep, in and out, as people came and went, and I felt guilty. I didn't want to be rude, but I had no control over my alertness the next few hours as the pain medication overtook me. I felt so shaky but didn't realize it was only me that felt shaky. I was nervous for others to hold her, thinking they were the ones shaking. Pictures taken at the time so easily show a sleepy smile upon my face as I held her those first few hours.

It's over is all I could think. *We made it.* I have my baby, maybe not necessarily the day or way I would have planned, but we are both here, healthy and alive. And now, with the c-section behind me, I couldn't be more ready to go home and begin life as a mother of three.

Two

I am that girl who from childhood always wanted things perfect. Or at least seemingly perfect.

New shoes at the age of 3? I didn't want to wear them for fear of getting the bottoms dirty. Although they were pretty and new, I couldn't enjoy them — the fear of 'ruining' them held me back. And just the bottoms, mind you.

Hand in hand with my dad, I was only going for a short walk up the street to see my grandma. I wasn't asked to walk in the rain or the mud, no. It was a beautiful summer day and we were walking on asphalt for about 30 whole steps. But I had a face full of tears under my huge glasses as I refused to wear a pair of new shoes I was given. I didn't want to mess them up. I would rather keep them looking perfect in their box — no evidence of being worn or used.

Life to me feels best if it's in an ordered fashion. I like things to be clean and just so. And for what I could control, life would be that way. But after being pregnant with my first baby and having him at 36 weeks, I found myself holding him during screaming episodes of acid reflux and food allergies … let's just say it wasn't the way I had envisioned it. So many other moms around me made all this newborn baby stuff look easy. And there I was, holding an infant whose skin seemed to break out regardless of what I ate, who cried for hours and crawled up my chest and neck with his nails after a feeding. My husband, whose motto in life is "It's fine," would look at me during those episodes in the middle of the night and would realize that in these moments everything wasn't fine. We were exhausted and clueless and, at times, felt desperate.

As a first-time mom, I initially thought this was normal. I thought life with a newborn was supposed to be exhausting, hard, and stressful with lots of crying from both of us. I didn't know any different. After losing more weight than I should have in trying to tailor my diet to suit the needs of my baby's belly, I realized that I might not be able to continue nursing him anymore. We had made it until 11 months, and I felt as though I had nourished him the best that I could. It seemed in the best interest for the both of us that he should be weaned. It broke my heart — that perfectionist in me wanted to keep going, but I wasn't able to figure out how to nourish myself. Many had mentioned their worries over my health, and I, too, had come to the point of being concerned. I had some peace that he was almost a year and was on some solids.

What my first year of baby-food-allergies and being a mommy did teach me, though, was to be grateful for the easy little nurslings that my second and third children were. Both Grant and Arianna, each born at 39 weeks, latched on immediately, and we never had a problem nursing. I was also cautious around any form of milk, cheese, etc. — pretty much anything that I thought might cause a reaction. Though there were some minor issues, having my next two children was easy. Maybe I was more experienced, maybe it was because they weren't born early. Whatever the reason, I was able to enjoy them more and I was so glad that they didn't have to experience what their brother did.

Being a mom of boys, I had gotten used to cars and trucks and the oh-so-unexciting clothes for which I would shop. Now holding and rocking a little Miss, I was excited to see how we would be able to bond as mother and daughter and have a lifelong relationship even after she was grown and married.

Any mom who nurses knows that in the early months, the provision of food that comes from your body for that new baby is a full-time job. Nursing and nursing again, around the clock, with not much of a break in between. And if there *is* a break, and you have other children, you are usually helping them, preparing some sort of meal, or anything that might resemble a meal, or considering the possibility of that luxury called a three-minute shower.

Oh, the decisions that seem so important in the first few months postpartum. Shall I shower? Shall I eat? Maybe I shall sleep. At this point, survival mode is the name of the game. And amidst it all, there are those sweet precious moments of holding, loving, and just staring at your new baby. I would sit there and just stare in awe and wonder that this little human, so dependent upon me for survival and needs and nourishment in every way, was created inside of me. The whole thing is completely above my ability to comprehend and understand. I would sit in awe and dream of who she may become and what life will be like as she grows — all the ups and downs we will experience together.

I was blessed with three children, healthy and strong. Every need was met in our lives. And then my mind would travel back in time to the days when it was only Preston and me.

I remember the pain I felt in desiring more children — in fact, I had believed it to be my calling to have many more children — but at the time it didn't seem possible since my monthly cycles had become so inconsistent.

It was just about fall, a year and a half after Preston was born. Walking around the county fair with our family, I tried to be present and engage in all the things our son was experiencing. We were surrounded by food, animals, tractors — it was always a time to meet and catch up with those we hadn't seen for so long. It was a special time of the year within our community. I wanted to enjoy all these things, but my mind was elsewhere.

I received a text from a friend who shared the great news that she was expecting her second child. We had had the joy, along with a few other friends, of sharing our first pregnancies at the same time. It was wonderful to have friends to experience this new phase of life with. Some of us had morning sickness, some didn't even know they were pregnant for two months. We got huge together. We went to each other's baby showers. We were celebrating *life* — it was truly good fun. We got to make those phone calls to each other when our own babies were born. It was so fun to receive the news that a dear friend had delivered her baby. But now, they were all pregnant for the second time … and I was not.

Life is not a race. Comparing my life to theirs wasn't right. But I couldn't help but feel 'behind' as they continued growing their families. My greatest desire and calling was for children, but with very random cycles it seemed nearly impossible. I had never struggled with inconsistency in my body before — it felt foreign to me, and I didn't understand. The three-year-old me had in her mind what was just right, just perfect. Any deviation from that made me feel frustrated, like my plans were being ruined and taken off the course of life I had planned many years ago.

Don't we all have those thoughts? Of how our children should be spaced according to our preferences and desires? I had zero trouble conceiving my first. The first month we thought about being *open* to a baby I had a positive test. It was easy. I almost felt like I, again, was in control. Something I wanted had happened on my timetable — I was comfortable and felt in charge.

From the outside, my family unit of three at the time looked pretty put together. We were young, had just built a new beautiful home, and had no worries or concerns. We seemed to have it all. But there was that part inside of me that ached as the one thing I wanted, the *one* thing I dreamed of, wasn't happening.

And then there was that ugly emotion no one likes to admit they experience from time to time. Jealousy. It would easily creep into my heart before I even realized what it was. It was yucky. It was messy, and I had to fight it continually. I didn't want it inside me, yet at the most unexpected times it would surface. That ugly, bad jealousy that would turn my happy feelings for others into sadness for myself. Ick. I would find myself ashamed that my heart would even go there.

I spent a lot of time trying to balance the desires I had for more children with the jealousy that would so easily creep in. It doesn't feel good to feel jealous. I had to fight it. So often we forget the blessings in our own lives and instead crave what others have, or seem to have. I think it's because I felt desperate for something I couldn't make happen. No matter how hard I tried to figure things out, no matter what options I looked to, the thing I wanted most and didn't have became a kind of obsession. I wanted to be happy for anyone who possessed this thing I didn't have — I wanted to celebrate with them for their gift. I might be able to fake it and smile and wish them well. But then I would start to dislike them.

There was a burning inside. A burning that I can't have what I want. And since I am not a superhero or some kind of super human, since I don't have super abilities, I couldn't change any of it. And it just plain stinks. And it's a sad admission. It was really a time for God to root out this yucky place inside my heart. It needed to go.

I always imagined myself being able to have a baby when I wanted to. And truthfully I felt like my plans for our life were being spoiled. My schedule, my timeline, was not being followed, and it bothered me. Though I didn't understand what was happening in my body, I eventually decided the best way to keep moving forward was to be thankful. Yes, I had to decide.

Sure, I had crying moments. I definitely had my moments through prayer, asking God *why*. I had my angry, I-don't-understand moments. But I decided to love the life that God had given *me* and enjoy the child God had given *me*. I tried not to look around so much at other people. I realized that had never brought me much good.

But drawing closer to God brought me great relief. Reading the Word, writing down the Word, chewing on the Word, and letting it absorb into my heart gave me peace and hope. I learned that He is good. That I would trust Him not based on what I saw — for we live by faith not by sight. I learned that I would trust Him because He is good. He is, no matter what things may disappoint me or hurt me. I am so grateful that through it, He showed me more of Himself. He *wants* to show us great and mighty things, but I needed to quiet my heart enough to hear His voice.

The little girl who, with tears and big glasses, had her own idea of perfect, neat, and clean decided to trust God. What other choice was there, really? Through the constant conflict of the yearning to expand our family and trying to be content with what I had been given, I kept walking. Kept moving.

Three

She was trying to convince me to go shopping. It's something I hadn't done often, as I was consumed with taking care of Preston and figuring out his food needs. Then after moving into our new home, there always seemed to be more important things keeping me occupied.

"Let's go shopping," Kate, one of my best friends and a roommate from college, said. "Chris won't mind. I will help you pick out some new clothes." Kate and her husband Chris had come from out of state for a visit to our new home. We always cherished our times together, especially since they were few. We were able to instantly pick up from where we last were.

"Are you sure?" I asked, picking up Preston and holding him on my hip.

It was early in the morning, raining and dreary outside. Kate and I were in the kitchen, cleaning up after breakfast, while Chris was upstairs in the guestroom. As it was a weekday, Ben was at work.

"Yes, he can go to Starbucks and work on his computer while we shop. He won't care at all. Come on, it will be fun!" She had the brightest, most hopeful eyes. And she looked at me with a smile. My great friend. She always genuinely cared for others and put the focus on them. Her heart was definitely not focused on herself or her own behalf. She was constantly reaching out to those around her and trying to meet their needs.

With hesitation, I agreed to go on the shopping trip. Kate was a great dresser, super pretty with her blonde hair and blue eyes. She was so fun to be with, and we would always talk about real things going on in our lives. I knew I would probably walk away with some wonderful, beautiful clothes that she'd pick out for me. But more than that, I knew I would walk away refreshed and encouraged. I knew her positive spirit would rub off on mine.

We loaded up the car with stroller in tow, dropped off Chris, and had ourselves a nice little spree, to say the least. Feeling depressed from Preston's health challenges, and it being 18 months with irregular cycles — with no other pregnancy in sight — I hadn't done much shopping for myself. It was nice to be with Kate, who focused on helping me and picked out so many new clothes, convincing me all the while that I was worth it. We spent a lot of time shopping, and I returned with several bags of very beautiful items that would provide a nice new wardrobe for months to come.

At home, we started to make dinner, and Ben arrived from work. While eating, we enjoyed one another's company and discussed our families, our daily lives, and our dreams and plans for the future. After cleaning up a bit, Kate and I drifted to the dining room and ended up talking alone. We sat on our cream-colored carpeted floor as I showed Kate health results I received from a natural doctor. I was working with him in attempts to strengthen my body in a natural, non-medicinal way. The results weren't a diagnosis of any kind, but it was more of a test to show any deficiencies I had and how my body was processing food. The results showed I was lacking many vital nutrients.

"It's not true," she said, flipping through the stapled papers, her eyes skimming over the various results. "You are healthy." She stared, refusing to accept what was recorded on the report. She kept looking at it and telling me that it wasn't true.

"You eat healthy — you are fine," she said encouragingly, from her compassionate and loving heart.

And I wanted very much to believe that everything was fine. But I just hadn't been feeling right. I was tired — weak, run down.

We talked some and then returned to the living room with Ben and Chris. I sat on the floor beside Ben as he rested comfortably on our tan leather couch.

I always loved being with Kate and Chris. As pastors at a large, thriving church, they were people who wanted to know what was really going on and had a heart to listen to you. They drew out the deep parts of people with caring questions and listening ears and hearts.

"I just want to have more babies," I said to them with tears. "I feel like that's what God wants me to do, but how can I? This doctor says I am deficient in so many nutrients, and since having Preston, my body feels so different, so weak."

I am sure they could sense the discouragement within me. It wasn't hard to spot. I had felt my entire life my calling was to be a wife who served the Lord, love my husband, and be a mom.

A career and the working world had no pull on me. After all, I attended college and did my best there. But I knew I wasn't there to prepare for a career. It just was not in my heart at all.

Without any words of advice or counsel, Chris came closer to us and said, "Let's pray."

I closed my eyes and rested for a moment in the comfort of their words.

As they prayed for us, I don't remember exactly what was said, but I do remember I felt extremely valued and cared for by our friends. They were always so supportive and encouraging — not just to us, but all people they encountered. It was their very nature.

After they finished praying, Chris looked at me. "I don't know what is in this chapter, but I just saw *Isaiah 54* in my head while we were praying." He sat on the couch as he spoke. He seemed so sincere — he really felt like he had a word for us, but wasn't sure what it was.

Ben reached over and picked up the Bible sitting on our glass coffee table. I sat there listening, staring at the carpet while Ben opened to that chapter and read:

"'Sing, barren woman, you who never bore a child; burst into song, shout for joy, you who were never in labor; because more are the children of the desolate woman than of her who has a husband,' says the Lord. 'Enlarge the place of your tent, stretch your tent curtains wide, do not hold back; lengthen your cords, strengthen your stakes. For you will spread out to the right and to the left; your descendants will dispossess nations and settle in their desolate cities … Though the mountains be shaken and the hills be removed, yet my unfailing love for you will not be shaken nor my covenant of peace be removed,' says the Lord, who has compassion on you … I will make your battlements of rubies, your gates of sparkling jewels, and all your walls of precious stones. All your children will be taught by the Lord, and great will be their peace … you will have nothing to fear."

With tears flowing from my eyes, I try to hold back the sobbing I felt welling up. I looked at Ben, his eyes red and face wet. Could this be? Is this truly from the Lord for me? I looked at them with questioning eyes wanting to understand more, but none of us did. I later wrote in my Bible next to Isaiah 54: "From Chris 8/19/07."

This became what I held onto in those moments where my dream and calling felt unattainable. Those times I became so discouraged but chose not to make my true feelings known to anyone. Whenever I struggled, I turned back to these words, believing in my heart that God had a great plan, even if I didn't know it or understand.

Four

I sat there looking at the words written before me. The Bible open on my bed while I rested. I reflected on who God said He is. I read His words that also said *who I was in Him*.

It was naptime. Preston was sound asleep, and I had quiet moments to myself with God, wanting wisdom and strength from Him. Even in my growing-up years, I would spend a lot of time alone, in my room with the door shut and my Bible open. Being an introvert, those times gave me what I needed to recharge and be able to go through my day. I was always eager to steal away time alone. Being with God left me feeling refreshed.

Still very much wanting another baby and very much holding onto Chris's words of encouragement, I came to a time when my periods and cycles just completely stopped. And they continued in that pattern for the next several months. When October arrived, I decided to make an appointment with a gynecologist and to have bloodwork done.

She was helpful and sincere as she looked at me with her strawberry blonde hair and white coat over her dress clothes. She sat next to me and explained what was necessary for me to do.

"You really need to take this. It will jumpstart a period. The risks of not having a period this long could in fact increase your chance for developing cancerous cells. Your bloodwork shows that nothing within your hormones seems to be off. Here is the prescription."

Sitting there, I struggled to believe she didn't have any answers for me either. Except medicine. But no true reason why my body wasn't seeming to function correctly.

I left her office on that cold day, got in the car, and eventually shared with Ben her warnings and advice. *Do I take this? Is this what God wants me to do?*

With much conversation and prayer, Ben and I decided we didn't feel led to take the medicine. I didn't have peace about it, but would just trust the Lord to give me direction. He had already spoken to me earlier in the previous months that I would indeed conceive again and have a baby before fall the next year. One might ask, "How did He tell you that?" And to answer: it was in prayer — an overwhelming sense of God's presence upon my soul.

"OK, God, you say I'm going to have a baby. Now I don't even have a cycle. Am I completely crazy here? What is going on?" These were my thoughts continually for the next few months. I started to doubt myself. I questioned myself. I questioned God. And I didn't let anyone know what the Lord had shared with me — it was just too precious to be talking about with anybody. It was in my heart. It was intimate words from my Heavenly Father.

Deep in prayer one night while drifting to sleep, I dreamed of going to talk to my pastor to ask him how I could trust the Lord in this. I felt as though God spoke to me and gave me words to cling to, that I would have another baby. But if that were the case, where were my cycles? How was I supposed to know if I really did hear from God? I was going to tell the pastor the words I felt were from Him. And I wanted to ask him how to interpret it all. I wanted to ask him if I was ... crazy.

In the dream I was just ready to walk into his office, and I stopped to hear the words, "Just believe, Mark 10:27."

There was no face to the voice, it was not the pastor's voice. I immediately woke up.

Wait. Wait! I wanted to hear more. But it was gone. The dream was over. Mark 10:27. I had no idea what that verse was. I drifted back to sleep.

Upon waking the next morning, I remembered my dream and opened my Bible.

Mark 10:27: "And Jesus looked at them and said, 'With man this is impossible, but not with God; all things are possible with God.'"

What in the world? Was this for me? I sat there, Bible in hand, just staring at the words. Surely I didn't come up with this on my own? I didn't know this verse by heart or from memory.

With MEN this is impossible. IMPOSSIBLE. IMPOSSIBLE.

BUT. NOT. WITH. GOD.

WITH. GOD. ALL THINGS ARE POSSIBLE.

OK. I sat there — stunned. It's true. Nothing, absolutely nothing, is impossible with God.

I will say it again. Nothing is impossible with God. Nothing in my life, nothing in yours.

With man, yes, many, many things are impossible. But right there it said that NOTHING is impossible with Him. I decided to hold onto that truth as I waited for days, that turned into weeks — then Thanksgiving, then Christmas. I held onto His promises despite what my physical body was doing and what my earthly eyes were seeing.

Still with no cycle, I decided to take some natural supplements to help. In December of that same year, I finally got a cycle and found out a few days before my birthday in January that I was indeed pregnant with a baby due in the fall, exactly what I felt the Lord had told me.

God fulfilled His promise to me. Had I listened to the doctor against my conviction, I most likely wouldn't have been pregnant at that exact time, which is what I felt God impress upon my heart earlier in 2007.

I was overjoyed at the idea of having another baby. But more overjoyed to see how the Lord carried me through a hard time in my life. He spoke to me through prayer, through people, and through His Word. I was more overjoyed to see that I had truly heard from the God of the universe. That what I thought He spoke to my heart He actually DID speak to my heart. My baby would be born at just the time the Lord told me he would be. I had conversed with God, the Creator — and I felt His blessing heavily on my life.

Five

"You can't do it. The risks are too high. We wouldn't want your uterus to contract," Dr. Hale said to me.

"Well, could I possibly just go into labor naturally before the c-section?" I responded. "With my first two babies, I did go into labor on my own, and my last baby I ended up coming to the hospital on the day I was scheduled for a c-section. I had so much anxiety. Aren't there certain hormones that change when you go into labor that help you bond better with the baby? Could I just go into labor first? I would feel so much better about that."

My heart raced as I spoke these words, asked these questions. Here I was, requesting the doctor change things for me. Challenging the way they do things. Why can't I just be quiet and do it their way? It's so much easier. I knew it was a mouthful, but I needed to lay out all my questions, all my thoughts. I patiently waited for his answers.

He looked at me from his chair as I sat on a table covered with white sterile paper. He, dressed in a white shirt and tie, and me, in my black yoga pants, trying to look presentable even though I was still feeling morning sickness at 14 weeks. It was all I could do to sit there, calm, and try not to let the churning in my stomach overtake me. The fact was: I needed to have this conversation with my doctor. It was of the utmost importance to me. I was focused. I had a pretty good idea of what he might say, but I wanted to give him the benefit of the doubt — a chance to share his views and perspective.

"No, there aren't any hormonal changes that make you bond better with your baby. And we wouldn't even want you to go into labor. The risk is too great. And no, we can't wait for you to go into labor because if everyone did that we would be having c-sections at 3 in the morning. It's hard to get everyone involved there when they need to be. It would need to be scheduled." He was very matter-of-fact.

"Well, you DO allow VBACs here, right?" I asked, heart still racing. I looked down at my hands in my lap. "I mean, if it's not safe for me, it's probably not safe for me. But let's say for a mom who has had one c-section … you do VBACs here, right?"

I sat there desperate for his answer. I knew it, but I had to hear it directly from him. Although glad to be having the conversation, I disliked it immensely. It was quite uncomfortable. I think it would probably be easier to ask all these questions had I had one or two c-sections in the past. But with three, I just had this feeling, an intuition, that my doctor wouldn't even see it as an option for me. The hospital just started "allowing" VBACs, and that was on a case-by-case basis — rumor was after only one c-section. I had not even planned on discussing this with him, but was actually encouraged by someone I trusted to share my feelings with him and be open about what I wanted.

"Yes, but that was mostly instituted for the Amish women. Let's say a woman comes in and has five kids and the sixth is breech. We do a c-section. We figure she is going to keep having children, so we might as well have a VBAC with her next time. Plus, you've never had a vaginal delivery before, so your chances are low."

"OK," I said.

I had just done so much reading about all the hormones that change and take place in birth.

I sat there stunned and saddened that this was the information he was giving me. I had so much respect for him, but for him to say that there are no hormonal changes in labor? Isn't it obvious there are?

My chances of a successful vaginal birth were low? Based on what? That I had not had the opportunity to try before? What about a first-time mother? Are her chances low also?

So many thoughts flooded my mind — mostly disappointment, that there was no possibility for me to deliver my baby with this doctor and hospital, that I don't agree with the facts he shared with me, and that I would be on a difficult road to find someone to support me during my pregnancy.

But hearing his opinion and recommendation for me, that journey was confirmed now — I knew I had some work to do.

My appointment ended. I knew then I wouldn't continue to receive care for my pregnancy at this office. The doctor had always been kind to me and valued life, considering every unborn baby precious, but no way in my heart did I feel as though consenting to a fourth c-section was what I was supposed to do. There had to be other options. I just didn't know what they were. I knew people had home births. I saw many benefits and advantages to that, but didn't feel led to that with my circumstances.

After the birth of my second child, I had already tried to find someone who would support me in having a vaginal birth for the next one. I could find no one and consented to another cesarean after many phone calls. I had already tried this in the past. But I knew I would leave no stone unturned.

I would have to dig deeper. I was willing to go wherever God would take me if someone would support me.

The very next day I was on the phone, calling various doctors in the area. The next few weeks I spent hours, literally, on the phone. And at times, I would wonder who I was even talking to.

"Hello, Dr. Lehman's office. How can I help you?

"Hi, my name is Jaimie Schrock. I was calling to see if the doctor there assists mothers who are pursuing VBACs. I have had three c-sections and am looking for a doctor to support me through a trial of labor."

"Ummmm, I'm not sure. Let me check." I could hear her muffled voice as her hand covered the phone, "Joan, does Dr. Lehman do VBACs? I don't know. Someone's called asking."

Then, she was back on the phone: "What is a VBAC?"

At this point, I was almost speechless. I had that sick-to-my-stomach feeling — the receptionist who works for an OB/GYN doesn't even know this. I explained it to her, and she told me she would get back to me.

No really, that's OK, I thought. But I let her take my information down in hopes that the doctor does indeed work with moms interested in VBACs and that this receptionist was simply uneducated.

Call after call I was told no. The doctors cannot assist me considering my situation. I had called every doctor and hospital in the area that I could get a phone number for. Everyone.

Upon the recommendation of my good friend Michelle, I called a local doula, Katie, whom I had never met before.

She seemed upbeat, positive, and extremely helpful — and she didn't even know who I was!

I told her my situation and said, "Do you think I am crazy for wanting this? Is it even a possibility?"

"No, you aren't crazy. This is a totally reasonable desire. I know of a local mom who had a vaginal delivery after three c-sections. If she's OK with it, I can get her number for you and you can talk to her." *That would be wonderful.* I could not wait to connect with this rockstar mom who has birthed her baby naturally after three c-sections. I wanted to talk with her. Like yesterday.

"Also, I really think you should call Dr. Sheffield. I think he'd be very open to your situation."

I sat on my kitchen floor. Cell phone and pen in hand, doodling on paper as I listened to her.

"Really? But I already called the hospital, and they said they only do VBACs after one, possibly two c-sections."

Katie convinced me. "Call the office and make the appointment. When you are sitting down with him, tell him your situation. I think you might have a good chance with him."

At her recommendation, I called the office, explaining I needed a new doctor and would like to meet with Dr. Sheffield. I was excited to secure an appointment even if they didn't know exactly why.

I sat in disbelief. My first appointment with this doctor was made. I would get to present my case, and he might actually listen. I got excited as my mind played through our forthcoming conversation. My heart racing, my hands sweating — I was so thankful.

Days later, when I had my next opportunity to make some calls, I decided to call my local ICAN (International Cesarean Awareness Network) chapter leader.

ICAN is a national organization whose mission is to improve maternal-child health by reducing preventable cesareans through education, supporting cesarean recovery, and advocating for vaginal birth after cesarean (VBAC).

"First, dear, you need to correct your language," the chapter leader told me. "No one lets you have a VBAC. You don't go into an appointment asking them to 'let' you. You ask if they would be willing to support you in a trial of labor."

What? I am the one in control, not the doctor? I stood there next to my kitchen counter, holding the phone, writing down her words. *Quoting* her words, so I would know how to talk to whichever doctors I'd speak to.

"This is YOUR birth, YOUR baby, YOUR body."

I began to think on her words. I had never heard this before. Usually the doctor tells the patient what to do, not the patient interviewing the doctor for the job. It was all new to me. I just stood there. Thinking and rethinking. And it made complete sense, but I hadn't thought this way before. Why was I just now realizing how true this is and how backward our system is?

"Well, OK." I said, still not convinced I could even do that. "Do you know of ANY doctor who would consider my situation?"

"The one doctor I would suggest is Dr. Marks. If anyone would do it, it would be him."

She gave me his information, and a couple other possible recommendations if that didn't work out. She also explained that a homebirth would be possible, but only under the supervision of a highly trained, experienced midwife.

Still standing there. Still feeling morning sickness. But I now had a full page of notes with powerful ways to express my desires with any future doctor. I had names and numbers — different possibilities. A priceless piece to my puzzle.

Once our conversation finished, I immediately called Dr. Marks' office, heart pounding, and was told he was on vacation. They would call me back.

And when I did receive that call, they asked to have my medical records faxed over from my previous surgical births. After many phone calls between my current hospital and Dr. Marks' office, and a few days of awaiting his response, I was told yes, he would be able to meet with me.

To say that I wanted to scream and shout would be an understatement. I had an appointment with the doctor who would most likely support me in this birth. I was almost in disbelief. Many hours invested in calling various offices, feelings of frustration mixed into that. I finally had some really great options on the horizon. The dream of the birth I wanted was a step closer to coming true.

I was overjoyed. Even though I had to wait a month, an appointment was set with Dr. Sheffield on a Wednesday and then with Dr. Marks on Friday of the same week. I felt confident that ONE of them had to say yes. After countless hours of work, I was getting somewhere.

The library and I became very close friends during that month. Any helpful book I could get my hands on. Any suggestions made to me that would further educate me, empower me, and give me the confidence I needed as I approached these two men and presented my wishes.

That month of waiting for those two special days was filled with all the normal mom stuff I was doing. I worked with my children on their schooling, I did my daily tasks to run our home life, all while struggling with feelings of nausea. Though I was very present in all that was before me, underneath my mind was fixed upon my baby and the birth. Those thoughts of an unmedicated, natural birth never left me. It was a deep desire, for many reasons, to birth my baby the way I was created to.

I hadn't had those typical "first moments" with any of my babies. I didn't get to hold them right away, look into their eyes, nurse them. Someone else pulled them from my body, took them away to weigh, measure, assess, and dress them, only to return them to me an hour or more later. I did not get to experience labor to the fullest extent and push out my baby, with all the supporting hormones that accompanied the process. My babies were given to me while I was heavily medicated and unable to fully take in those precious moments — the beginning of our relationship. And, oftentimes, there were many other people present when I met my children for the first time. I wasn't able to comfort them and love them as they transitioned from the inside of my body to a world that was so stimulating and unfamiliar to them. I wanted this *badly* this time around. I knew that having many c-sections only increased the possibility of serious complications. I desired more children after this. And if that were to happen for me, I did not want to keep having them in an operating room.

As my baby grew inside, the cells of that little body were growing and changing and developing, I was growing and changing too. I was learning to trust God each day, each step of the way. In the waiting, I worshiped Him through song and thought. I prayed. I surrendered my fears to Him. I rested in who He said He was. My love for the Lord grew, and I longed for how He would work in my life.

Six

"Why do you even want to do this?" my close friend Stacy asked me as we watched our children play together.

We were at the park — we had it to ourselves. The weather was trying to break and we wanted to take advantage of it. It had been a long winter, so the mild temperatures that day were very inviting. Looking up, I saw my youngest on the swing, sloshing her boots back and forth through the wet mud puddle below her.

I knew the conversation would come up at some point, but I didn't think it would be today.

My throat was suddenly in a knot. I tried to hold back the tears. I wished she would just *get* me... It was hard for me to explain to someone why. There were too many reasons.

Without waiting for my reply, she said, "This is so dangerous. And it will take up a lot more of your time, driving so far for your appointments."

I could hear it in her voice. Annoyance, confusion … she didn't understand where I was coming from.

She was right. If I were to stay with my local doctor, I was only 15 minutes away — very convenient. But should Dr. Marks work out, I would be driving an hour one way for each appointment. But it was a sacrifice I was willing to make.

"Statistically it's actually MORE dangerous for me to have

another c-section," I said with a convincing tone in my voice. "And if I want to have more kids after this baby? Forget it — I won't if I have four surgeries. I can't do that. It's too much."

Thing is, I shouldn't have had to convince her, or anyone. I was telling the truth. But most people haven't spent the time to take a good look at the information. They are just accustomed to what most people do.

I had done so much research on the risks and benefits of VBAC versus c-section for my circumstances. Contrary to public knowledge, the American College of Obstetricians and Gynecologists actually suggests that most women with one or two previous c-sections be given the opportunity for a trial of labor. Why aren't most doctors telling women this? Instead, they state the risks involved. It's amazing the information we *aren't* given when we visit a doctor. And if we don't go digging around for it ourselves, our eyes remained blinded to the truth.

"Why would you want more kids? God's been good to you. You will have four. Girl, you'd be crazy to have more! No one does that anymore!" Her words were effortless — she had already made up *her* mind about my circumstances.

My eyes filled with tears. I only wished she — a friend I loved dearly — would understand my heart.

I wished *most* people in my life would understand my heart in this. But they didn't. People with whom I was close — people who were only acquaintances … most of them didn't know enough to really understand why I felt the way I did. I heard all kinds of responses:

"Well, if it were safe, they would let you do it."

"It's not about how you birth your baby as long as mom and baby are safe."

"Why do you want to do this again? Wouldn't it be easier if you just had surgery? Why would you want to go through labor when you can just go in and have the baby and not feel anything?"

"You are making this harder than it should be."

"Oh, I know a girl who had three sections. She can't have a vaginal birth. She's not allowed. I didn't even know you could have a vaginal delivery after a section." Confused look.

It was constant.

(And I would like to say, I had no hard feelings toward anyone's opinions. I knew if they had done the research like I did, they would be right there with me in it. Sadly, most pregnant women who desire a VBAC are left to field all kinds of opinions from the general public. It's not uncommon at all. Most believe it is dangerous, unwise, even negligent of a mother to desire this. Most don't understand why anyone would even choose to walk such a path. It seems easier and safer to have a repeat surgery. It's just the way our society is — it's how we've been molded to think. Unless you are faced with having to search for the facts, sadly they aren't easily found.)

Since I have been a people-pleaser since birth, I like to make people happy. I like it when they like me. I like it when things are smooth and there is no conflict. It's what I know and what is comfortable to me. I had never been a brave girl, ready to try new things. I even screamed on the Tilt-o-Whirl at the county fair as the rednecks stared, wondering what was wrong. Going against the grain, stepping out into the unknown, was just not part of my nature.

But this was different.

I cared. I wanted what was best for my family, my baby, myself. I did not see a fourth surgery being the best. I wanted to have a shorter recovery with three other children to care for afterward. I wanted by body to go through labor, for the baby to go through that labor, so we could bond with the healthiest outcome possible. I didn't want either of us to have drugs circulating in our systems, but rather natural hormones — as nature intended. I didn't want the routine antibiotics given after c-sections. I wanted the option of more children. If there was any part of me that believed a vaginal birth was more dangerous to myself or my baby, I would in no way seek it out. That would truly be irresponsible. But I wanted the best for all of us, for now and in the future, and I believed a VBAC was just that.

I wasn't seeking a certain experience. I wasn't trying to make myself "become a real mom" by delivering naturally. The thought never crossed my mind. My sole pursuit was to do what I felt was the absolute best option for my baby, myself, and my family.

I sensed a difference in my spirit, something new inside of me. I had to trust God. I had to seek pleasing Him, following Him, honoring Him, no matter what any person, acquaintance, or loved one wanted for me. Naturally I wanted their approval. I really did. But I knew my Father was saying, "Trust *Me*." I had to let go of what anyone thought, good or bad.

Day by day, minute by minute, I had to align my thoughts and emotions with what the Lord thought of me. And I knew as long as my heart was seeking Him, He was pleased.

Very quickly I learned to stop sharing with others what plans I was pursuing. I came to a place where, emotionally, I couldn't handle the questions, the confusion, or even the slight possibility that there might be a lack of support. It made my heart ache to even think about it. I determined that I didn't have to explain anything to anyone. Impressed upon my heart was the reality that the only one I really needed to please was the God of the universe. And I had to trust that He would lead and guide me. This path was something between me and Him, and I would listen to His voice alone.

In the month preceding my much-anticipated appointments, I spent a lot of time reading my Bible, praying, listening to sermons online, and singing my heart out in worship to Him.

I needed *encouraging* words when I was alone on my journey. And that is how I felt: alone.

I did speak with one mom once who had a vaginal delivery after three c-sections. And for that I'm grateful. But I didn't have one human being to hold my hand through the process, who understood my thoughts and my fears and questions. No one I knew personally had done this.

But … I knew *Him*.

And I knew He would not lead me where He wouldn't go. In fact, that's a perfect summation of how I felt. He, the Lord my

God, would not lead me where He would not go and would not be. I knew that I was ready to trust Him in a way that I never had before. I wasn't interested in others' opinions. I wasn't interested in others' feelings. I was bathing this birth in prayer. This was my journey, and I would rest in Him each day that we traveled together.

This birth was so important to me. It went far back to what I believe was my calling from God — that I would be the mother of many children. *Many*. That's a word that doesn't clearly explain a number other than meaning more than a few. Was *many* four? Was *many* five? Did it mean some birthed naturally and others through adoption? I didn't know, but it was my responsibility to do all I could to leave the door open to however *many* He wanted to bless me with.

It's why I was passionate. It wasn't just about this baby, but about the future of our family. And children aren't created to bless their mother or fulfill some need of mine, they are created to worship and serve the Lord Almighty and point others to Him.

Yes, I love my babies. Yes, I love the feeling of my baby inside, moving, kicking, squirming, living closer than they will ever be again to me in their lives — literally growing and living off my body. But it's much greater and grander than that. It's to serve the purpose of raising up strong leaders who love the Lord, serve Him, and make a difference in this world. This was not about me and my agenda. This was about how we are able to fit into God's grand plan. And because of that, a deep passion propelled me to keep moving, keep going, and not to take my eyes off of Him.

Seven

It was the middle of March, and so beautiful outside. Spring was starting to give us glimpses of herself. It was warm enough to go without a coat, but too cold for short sleeves. The weather in our area, though, can be so funny … with warm, sweet sun on Wednesday and snowing by the end of the week.

Nevertheless, the rays of sun matched the hope within my heart that my appointment with Dr. Sheffield would be fruitful.

He didn't know why I was coming, only that I was looking for a new doctor in the area. The doula who recommended him, Katie, suggested I don't "present my case" until I am seated in front of him.

On my drive to his office, a mere 10 minutes away, I fervently prayed that God would work in my favor. Ten minutes from home would be such a blessing compared to the hour-long drive I'd have if the doctor in the city instead would be the one to accommodate my wishes.

"What should I say?" I spoke into my cell phone. "What if he won't even want to talk to me because he doesn't know that I am pregnant … and what if he's mad?"

"No, he won't be," said Michelle, one of my very best friends. She recently had a VBAC with Dr. Sheffield. Our local hospital, where she previously delivered, once vaginally and once by c-section, wouldn't allow her a VBAC past 40 weeks. As a result, she had gone on a wild goose chase trying to figure out where she could deliver and what doctor would support her — all at the last minute. Dr. Sheffield was the one to help her.

"Just tell him you are pregnant and you wanted to talk with him directly and not the receptionist. He won't think anything of it!" She was reassuring.

Michelle had always been good for me. She was optimistic, go-with-the-flow — a no-worries kind of girl. I, on the other hand, prefer a schedule and order, and would often easily go into Worry Mode. She brought fun into my life, lots of laughing, yet was also able to be serious. Best of all: we shared a common desire for following Christ.

I was 18 weeks along. Just starting to get a little bump, which was also easily unrecognizable to anyone who didn't know about the great gift growing within me. I was just starting to feel the baby's movements — such a joy! With each pregnancy, as I experienced those first little flutters, I had realized how easy it was to forget what they felt like. It was so reassuring to know that the baby inside me was growing stronger and able to move, letting me know of his or her presence.

Michelle continued to counsel me until the moment I pulled into the office parking lot. I was very grateful she was a familiar voice of comfort to me on the other end.

"Well," I said," I should go. I'm here! And late!" I tried to be polite, but all I could think about was getting inside and getting that appointment started.

"OK, let me know what he says. I am praying for you."

Placing my phone in my purse, I left the car, and walking to the building I took a quick peek through the glass window of the office door … I pulled the handle (wet armpits and all) and walked in.

"Hi, I have an appointment with Dr. Sheffield."

"Yes, and your name?" said the smiling receptionist seated behind the desk at the window.

I gave her my information and sat down to fill out all the paperwork. Shaking and sweating and writing, I noticed everyone behind the desk seemed so laid back.

No one was in the waiting room but me. I had my Bible with me. I thought to try to read a little before I was called back, but I just couldn't concentrate. I continued filling out forms and felt sick to my stomach. Not from morning sickness this time, but from the nerves. What would he say? What would he think? Would I even have a shot at this?

No matter what the outcome, I just had a peace that the Lord would provide. Whether this doctor or someone else, I would find someone. I just knew it.

The nurse called me back after I turned in my paperwork, and she took down my weight and blood pressure.

"Well," she said, "your blood pressure is somewhat high."

Yes, of course it is!, I thought … just a little anxious, that's all. I smiled at her, not knowing what response she expected.

She proceeded to ask me many questions once we were in the assigned room, all the way down to, "When was your last menstrual cycle?"

She kept typing on her tiny tablet, and I paused before I answered — her back facing me as she sat at her desk.

"Um," I said, "November 9th." And yes, today is March 19. So that was, well, a long time without a period if you do the math.

She turned from her desk to look at me.

"Oh, your cycle's a little off? Yes, that happens sometimes." She looked down and resumed her typing only to stop and turn back to me again.

Another pause.

"You couldn't be pregnant, could you?" she asked with somewhat of a blank expression on her face.

"Well, yes. Actually I am."

There. Cat's out of the bag. Let's move on to the reason I'm here. Not so sure how she will respond, but there's no way I was lying.

"Oooohhh," she said, surprised, but then continued acting like it was no big deal.

Things might get a little awkward now, I thought to myself. But they didn't. Maybe she didn't know what to say, since usually you mention this kind of thing *before* the appointment.

We continued with the list of mandatory questions on her tablet — background, history, etc.

Once she left the room, my eyes scanned the Psalms, taking in any tidbits I could with my lack of focus.

A knock at the door — Dr. Sheffield entered. He was dressed

very nice, and he, too, was a smiling person like the rest of his staff.

He greeted me with a handshake as I stood respectfully to say hello.

After some small-talk chit-chat, he asked, "So, what brought you in today ... how can I help you?"

In my most confident voice, I shared with him the story of my previous pregnancies. And then, I popped the question.

"I am about 18 weeks along with my fourth baby. I am looking for a doctor who would support me through a trial of labor. I don't want to consent to another c-section and would like to have a vaginal delivery. I have thought about it, researched it, and I feel as though it's in the best interest of my health and my baby's. I believe it is best for my family. Is this something you could support me in?"

Relief overcomes me instantly. My words came out like I had wanted them to. Deep breath of relief. The hard part was over. I was faithful on my end. And now I could listen for his response.

Dr. Sheffield looked at me with sincere compassion in his eyes. "I understand why you would want this."

My thoughts are going faster than his words are coming out: Really? You, a doctor, can see why I would want to do this?

"I can see your reasoning. But unfortunately, I cannot help you. My medical malpractice insurance is not high enough, and there's no way they would let me."

"So even if you wanted to, you couldn't because of legal reasons?"

"Yes. There's no way I would be able to."

A knock at the door called him quickly to the labor and delivery floor of the hospital, and he promised he would be right back. It was nice of him to assure me of his return, but I had my answer.

A few tears fell from my cheeks after he left the room. I knew it was only another doctor to turn me down, but I had been hoping for an easy *yes*. I opened my Bible to try to find some comfort and prevent the impending heartbreak.

PSALM 8

LORD, OUR LORD,
HOW MAJESTIC IS YOUR NAME IN ALL THE EARTH!
YOU HAVE SET YOUR GLORY IN THE HEAVENS.
THROUGH THE PRAISE OF CHILDREN AND INFANTS
YOU HAVE ESTABLISHED A STRONGHOLD
AGAINST YOUR ENEMIES,
TO SILENCE THE FOE AND THE AVENGER.
WHEN I CONSIDER THE HEAVENS,
THE WORK OF YOUR FINGERS, THE MOON AND THE STARS,
WHICH YOU HAVE SET IN PLACE,
WHAT IS MANKIND THAT YOU ARE MINDFUL OF THEM,
HUMAN BEINGS THAT YOU CARE FOR THEM?
YOU HAVE MADE THEM A LITTLE LOWER THAN THE ANGELS
AND CROWNED THEM WITH GLORY AND HONOR.
YOU MADE THEM RULERS OVER THE WORKS OF YOUR HANDS;
YOU PUT EVERYTHING UNDER THEIR FEET:
ALL FLOCKS AND HERDS,
AND THE ANIMALS OF THE WILD, THE BIRDS IN THE SKY,
AND THE FISH IN THE SEA,

ALL THAT SWIM THE PATHS OF THE SEAS.
LORD, OUR LORD,
HOW MAJESTIC IS YOUR NAME IN ALL THE EARTH!

The door again opened, and he graciously returned to give me names of other doctors he thought might be able to help me. He explained that a maternal fetal medicine doctor might be my best option, and I briefly mentioned my upcoming appointment with one in the next two days. He also explained the risks of multiple c-sections to me, including *accreta*, which no one had ever taken the time to do with me.

"Placenta accreta is a general term used to describe the clinical condition when part of the placenta, or the entire placenta, invades and is inseparable from the uterine wall. Clinically, placenta accreta becomes problematic during delivery when the placenta does not completely separate from the uterus and is followed by massive obstetric hemorrhage leading to … hysterectomy, surgical injury to ureters, bladder bowel … Maternal death may occur despite optimal planning, transfusion management, and surgical care. The incidence of placenta accreta has increased and seems to parallel the increasing delivery rate" (ACOG Committee Opinion, Number 529, July 2012).

I was very impressed that he continued to talk with me even though he would not be able to help me. He also gave me the risks of having more c-sections, and that was something I had not been previously informed of either. I never knew these risks in the detail in which he explained them to me. Any risks I had knowledge of were because of my own research, never from a consultation.

He spent a lot of time and heard me. And for *that* I was quite thankful. As we ended the appointment and he went to leave the room, he turned around and looked me in the eye.

"I will be praying for you, that you find the right doctor."

Bam — tears again flood my eyes … all I could do was say, "Thank you."

I was disappointed when I left the office, but I was not surprised. A lot of people had said *no* to me over the phone, so I wasn't shocked. But it just hurt a little bit. It would have been a lot easier on my end to not have to keep looking and making appointments. It would have been easier to know who my doctor was. But I didn't.

And I had to keep trusting God. I had to keep listening, following, knowing He would lead me to the right one — the best one — for me.

Sending Katie the doula a text, I told her he wasn't the one. "Onward and upward," I typed.

I wasn't going to stop. I would find a doctor. I would be persistent. Even if it meant driving an hour, or two, or three. I felt such an assurance. I knew God wouldn't leave, wouldn't forsake. I knew He had put this on my heart.

I kept telling myself that God would have not just a good doctor, but the best one. And in the end, that's exactly what I got.

Eight

"I think I have most everything packed," I told Ben. Rushing around in our small apartment, tripping over kids and suitcases, I went through the mental checklist in my head hoping not to forget anything.

"Here's everything that can go in the car," I instructed. "The only things left are the food in the fridge and the coolers I can pack when I get back." I knelt down and tried to quickly put shoes on, grab my keys, and go.

We were getting ready to leave for West Virginia for a weekend cabin trip with Ben's side of the family, but only after my morning appointment in the city to meet with Dr. Marks. I was headed there alone while Ben stayed with the kids. This was the last doctor with whom I had an appointment set. Other names still remained on my list, but I wanted to wait and see how this appointment would go.

I shut the door to the apartment and drew in a deep breath of the cold air. It was early, and snowy, in fact, and very quiet. Relief filled me. I would be alone and have time to think — and just *be*. I had looked forward to that.

Morning sickness came over me at times, more often than I would have liked. But I did my best to look somewhat presentable on the outside, so I had gotten dressed in an actual pair of jeans and a long black babydoll sweater and black boots. I knew appearances shouldn't matter, but I wanted to put my best foot forward, so I skipped the yoga pants this time around.

Green smoothie in one hand, water in the other, and toting my driving directions, purse, and cell phone, I was off to the city — literally passing a couple of free-range chickens as I left the driveway. I, the girl from the country, was on her way to the city.

I was a little nervous making the drive alone — I don't have the greatest sense of direction. But it was the best scenario for the situation, so I prayed and prayed on my way that God would help me and bless my time there. I tried to imagine what the office might look like, and how the appointment might go. It was something I had played over and over in my mind anyway. I tried to calm myself down — I didn't want my blood pressure to go up and give a bad reading my very first time there.

After the 60-minute drive on the highway, I found the parking garage and made my way to the elevator, to the second floor. My heart skipped when the doors opened and I walked down the halls, looking for the correct signs. I passed nurses and ladies with bellies, many of whom seemed friendly, who would smile, but who were also very much focused on where they were going.

The atmosphere was a little different from the good old farm area I was used to. My scenery at home consisted of fields, cows, and people mostly of the same color. The people in the city were diverse. Beautiful browns ... people with lighter skin and very dark hair and eyebrows. All colors, all kinds. So many different cultures and backgrounds represented. I mean, I could have been wearing a cowboy hat — I'm sure I seemed different as well. But this wasn't just an OB, but a Maternal Fetal Medicine doc. Many women came here to get the best care.

We were all pregnant, of course, but our circumstances were many. For me, it was to seek a VBAC, and I could think of nothing else.

There were two waiting areas within the office. I was confused about where to go and what I was supposed to be doing. I had trouble understanding the receptionist — she spoke with a heavy accent. There were SO many people there, and it was SO big compared to what I was accustomed to in my small town. It was enough to make me feel out of place and self-conscious.

Regardless, I sat down, commenced my wait, and opened up my copy of a well-known birth book, Ina May Gaskin's *Guide to Childbirth*, trying to educate myself while my heart raced and my mind wandered. I hoped my words would come out right when I was in front of the doctor.

"Remember this, for it is as true as true gets: Your body is not a lemon. You are not a machine. The Creator is not a careless mechanic. Human female bodies have the same potential to give birth as well as aardvarks, lions, rhinoceri, elephants, moose and water buffalo. Even if it has not been your habit throughout your life so far, I recommend that you learn to think positively about your body" (page 142).

Reading about the mind-body connection, I knew I had work to do. Being around people in my vulnerability made me nervous. I mean, I like my privacy. I am a private person. I knew that in childbirth privacy goes right out the window.

It was too hard for me to wrap my mind around what I had just read. I filed it away in my brain, waiting for another time where I would be more comfortable or ready to dive into the topic with myself.

"Miss Jaimie," the nurse said from the opened door in the waiting room.

I closed my book and quickly grabbed my things, hands trembling. Instantly I went from somewhat relaxed to nervous again. I wished I could control my anxiety better. I said a quick "hello" to the nurse who had just called me.

There was a small room on one side of the hallway that held a scale and blood pressure machine. I sat down to have my vitals checked and chit-chatted about the things you chit-chat about when you don't know someone well — to make it less awkward than complete silence.

Once I was settled in an examination room, a nurse came in to let me know the doctor would be in to see me in a few minutes.

"Do you think he would support me in a VBAC?" I asked her shakily.

I said it. I couldn't wait for the doctor. I felt impatient. I wanted to see if there was anything I could gather from *her* before laying it all out for the doctor.

"I don't know. He does that, but you will have to talk to him," she said quickly, right before she left the room.

That was all. No small talk. Just a quick answer. Well, at least she knew what a VBAC was. Maybe, *just maybe*, he would assist me.

It felt so different there. So foreign. The same doctor had delivered my first three babies. Doctors are professionals, who provide a service. But you never forget your children's actual birth days. You never forget who was there, what you were doing, what it all felt like. When choosing a provider and walking with them through this sacred time, it is easy for us to become connected to them.

I imagine most mothers understand. It's the most precious moment in your life when your child comes into the world. And even during the pregnancy, those nurses you see constantly at each appointment, even the front-desk staff … at this time in your life when you are growing a human being … it's sacred, and anyone who is along for the ride becomes part of the story.

But in that new office, I felt so out of place, so unfamiliar — I almost felt dishonest, as if going behind my doctor's back. He had been really wonderful to me. He was kind and always listened to my concerns. He wasn't emotional and seemed to always calm my fears and put me at ease — he was good for me. I had nothing against him, but I needed someone else, even if that meant leaving the safety of the familiar. Still, I felt insecure and unsure of the mood there — of the fast pace that seemed mirrored by the city.

A knock at the door.

A young girl in a white coat entered — a student.

"Hi. How are doing?" she asked, shaking my hand.

"Fine, and you?" I wanted to be polite with her. I understood she needed to learn, but I merely wanted, and needed, to talk to the man in charge. Not her. I didn't want her learning on *me*.

She sat down, and we proceeded thoroughly through my history, pregnancies, and deliveries. She smiled at me as she looked through her glasses, typing everything I said quickly onto her computer. I just wanted to get to the point. I may have felt differently any other time, but I knew my family was waiting for me back home so we could leave for our trip. I already felt bad enough making them wait, but I was hoping I wouldn't need to go over all of this info again once the doctor came in.

"OK, thank you. Dr. Marks will be in very soon." She smiled again as she left, and I returned a grin when I realized it was almost time to have the conversation I was there to have.

Picking up my book, I started reading again, and wondering again. Could I birth like the women in the book? Could I be one of them, one who goes through the natural process of bringing my baby into the world? Oh, I hoped so. I hoped for it more than anything else at the moment. It was so very important to me. More than any doctor, friend, or family member could know or understand.

To have come this far, was a victory in and of itself for me. I had pushed through with hours of research, conversations, phone calls, skepticism. I worked to get to where I was at that very moment. Pregnant, a homeschooling mother to three, a wife, living in an extremely small (and, albeit, temporary) apartment, experiencing morning sickness, aching for a different birth experience. I was driven, I was purposeful, and I was committed to walking in confidence as the Lord was guiding and directing me. My desire kept me motivated despite what any other person thought.

I was going for it.

A knock at the door again.

This time, it was the doctor.

Finally.

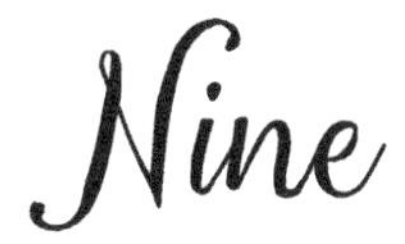

Sweating again, my heart racing while Ina May's *Guide to Childbirth* rested in my hands, I smiled and greeted him.

The doctor knelt down beside me as his student sat in the chair next to the computer.

"So," he said. "You are interested in a vaginal birth."

After saying *yes*, that was my purpose for coming, he then began to explain to me the risks — including rupture, death to the baby, or cerebral palsy. He also mentioned that the likelihood of those conditions was low, but that there were risks in involved.

"I want to make sure you are aware of the risks," he told me.

"Yes, I am fully aware of the risks. I know with anything there are risks."

I had done my homework. Everything he mentioned I already knew about. And I mean that without a hint of pride. This was my baby. I would do anything to protect the child inside me. Anything.

I had researched, scouring books and resources and studies online — anything I could get my hands on. I was not walking into this blindly. I would not have come this far, worked this hard, without concrete reasons about why I wanted a VBAC, *including* being well aware of things that could go wrong. But I was convinced that for me, they wouldn't. I *knew* that I knew this was the path I was to take.

We talked some more, and it almost seemed as though he was going to help me. It *seemed* like that's where he was going in the conversation ... when a nurse suddenly called him, and he ran out.

He apologized as he left, but I was thankful to see him running to labor and delivery. To me it meant he was a good doctor and was serious about his job.

So I sat there, still thinking: Could it be? Could he be the one to assist me in my pursuit of the birth I so desired?

He knew why I had come. And instead of being asked why I wanted what I did, I was able to hear his thoughts without having to present my case to him. He had already looked over my faxed-in surgical notes, and I was glad my purpose was now known.

I decided to check my phone — it had been going off since I sat down for the appointment. Four missed calls. From Ben, my sister, and my best friends, wanting to check how this ever-so-important meeting had gone.

"I think I'm in," I texted my friend Laura. "I think he's going to say yes. I think this is it."

I just sat there, stunned. How had it been so easy? He acted like it wasn't a big deal — almost as if explaining the risks were just part of his job yet not his greatest concern. After all my prayers, hours of research, and investment of time, money, and, above all, my heart, *this could be it.* My great desires could be fulfilled with his help.

When he returned to the room, he asked, "So, do you have

any questions?"

And I did. How long could I labor? ... How long could I labor from home? ... Would I have to be monitored continuously? ... How did he prefer to catch babies? ... and more.

To my great delight, his thoughts were pretty close to my own wishes and desires. Ninety-nine percent of what I wanted — though to some they might have seemed extreme — he was on board with.

"I am the closest doctor you will find next to a midwife," he said, sitting in his chair, typing notes into my file on the computer.

He looked at the book in my hands and remarked, "A friend gave me that book."

Wow. He had a book by Ina May, the mother of authentic midwifery. Was it too good to be true? I went from a doctor completely against even thinking about my trying a VBAC, to several doctors who tell me they won't even see me ... to this? Am I dreaming?

I was pleasantly perplexed: How, oh how, is this all coming together? It felt like a dream. There were so many women I had met online from all over the country who would have been extremely jealous to know what I had just discovered in this doctor. Women who had to fight to find a doctor, having put their hearts into their search, just as much as I had to, only to find no one to help, hearing the dreaded word *no*.

He asked to listen to the baby's heartbeat and mine. Which was still racing.

"So, I will be taking care of you from now on, is that OK?" he asked as I got down from the table.

I thought about the drive to the city, the foreign feel to me, breaking up with my doctor and leaving my small-town hospital, toting my kids with me to my appointments. Could I make this commitment? Could I really do it?

Why was I second-guessing myself? Why didn't I shout YES from the rooftops?!

"Yes," I said.

"Well, what I normally do," he said, "is write a letter to your doctor explaining that I will be taking over your care for the rest of the pregnancy. It would be best if you leave on good terms, as I am not a gynecologist, if you need to return to him for your needs and care regarding that."

I agreed to that, and also to having my 20-week ultrasound (already scheduled back home) with the results forwarded to Dr. Marks.

As he left the room, he said, "Get your phone. I'll give you my pager number. If you need anything, you can page me and I'll call you back. You don't have to go through the nurses. It's just easier this way."

I stood there, frozen. My phone. I hardly knew how to work my phone in that moment. How do I put a contact in? I tried to act like I knew what I was doing, fumbling with the keys. What kind of doctor gives his pager number to patients? I was going to get quality care from a doctor who truly wanted to help patients like me. I almost couldn't believe it, couldn't wrap my mind around it. *God*, I thought in my heart, *You truly did have the best plan for me. God, You are so good. You amaze me. Thank You. My heart already thanks You.*

I shake his hand and walk out of the room. Sweating. Relieved. Shocked. Confused. Excited. A million emotions running through my body and heart. The fight is — *over*.

I left his office that day in shock and disbelief. Pulling out of the parking garage and stopping at a light, I was immediately on the phone and sharing the news with those who cared the most.

I felt relief that the appointment was over. I was able to state my desires, approach another doctor, and leave knowing I was on my way to a VBAC. I didn't have to wonder anymore what this pregnancy would look like — I didn't have to keep making phone calls and try to find a provider. I didn't have to dream of whether or not I would be on the surgical table. My search was over. I was now able to focus on my preparation. My goal was very much in focus — I could press on toward what I felt I was called to do.

Driving home on the highway, my body just let go. Tears of joy burst from my eyes. Which turned into sobs. Crying and thanking God that He had answered my prayers. I was going to be able to have a trial of labor. I had found *the* doctor.

I felt the feeling you get when you run through the finish-line tape at the end of a race. I felt out of breath. Like I didn't have it in me to keep searching, keep running. Like I only had the energy for a few more steps before I collapsed.

But there I was, done running this leg of the race, and it

felt really good. It was worth the sweat, worth the pain I had to ignore, worth every *no* by so many others — worth the choice I made to not give up, to not back down. It was beyond the greatest relief and joy I had imagined.

God knew my deepest desires for this birth. He knew the kind of doctor I wanted, and needed, and it seemed as though this doctor would be more than I could have hoped or prayed for. God is good like that.

I love when He gives us not only what we ask for … but *more* than what we even knew we wanted in the first place.

My excitement overwhelmed me so much, in fact, that I got lost on my way home. Yes, lost! When I should have been quickly returning to make it home in time for our trip, I was lost. And without a navigation system on my old phone, my personal navigation system (my wonderful [sarcasm] sense of direction) failed me. I did my best, but my mistake ended up putting us behind an hour or so on our way to West Virginia. Ben was not happy about that part.

I, on the other hand, was on cloud nine. The happiest girl you ever did see. I was thanking the Lord for leading me to a great doctor. This thing that seemed impossible, that most people thought was dangerous, crazy, wrong, too hard, too much work … this thing was in sight for me. Praise the Lord. Praise the Lord.

Ten

"What do you think, Mommy?"

"I just have a feeling it's a boy," I said, putting on make-up and trying to find a shirt to fit my 20-week belly, "but I don't know." It was an awkward time: I wasn't looking pregnant, just rounder than usual. Maternity clothes didn't fit appropriately, and regular clothes looked slightly ridiculous. Good thing I wasn't getting ready for a fashion show.

"Well, I think it's a girl," said Arianna, as her big blue eyes looked up at me with such expectation and wonder.

I know most people think that would just be perfect, two boys and two girls, and you are set. The perfect little family.

Me, I didn't have a preference — I just wanted my baby to be growing properly and be thriving. I was thrilled to be having another child and almost felt like it was asking too much to desire a certain sex over the other. Given the responsibility to care for another child, which I had desired for so many years, I was incredibly thankful to be where I was. This was a gift enough for me. Whoever was in there, I would love and cherish that child knowing he or she would help make our family more complete.

Yes, I knew my little daughter would want a sister — that's what she wanted so badly this past Christmas — but I was trying to prepare her in case there was a little baby boy on the way. She really had her heart set on a sister, and I didn't want her to be totally disappointed.

"I really just have a feeling it's a boy. Another boy would be fun, wouldn't it?" I asked her as I did my hair. I had finally been feeling better — almost normal! It felt good to have the energy and strength to put on some make-up and do my hair.

"Well, I want a baby sister," Arianna said matter-of-factly. And what little girl doesn't? Someone to play dolls with, have tea parties, do each other's hair. The fun girly stuff. I can't imagine a little girl not wanting a sister.

Ben was on his way home from work, and we would soon be on our way to my 20-week ultrasound appointment with my original doctor.

It was our chance to look at our baby in great detail. The spine, the organs, the heart. I knew I should have been excited for the appointment, but I had overwhelming anxiety wondering if everything was OK. I'd love this baby no matter what, even if the doctor found something that was seemingly imperfect. But, you know? We *do* want that. We want the best and easiest life for each of our children. And if there's a health issue, it can be difficult and harder on them and on us.

It was a big day. I wanted to trust God. I wish I had enough faith to keep my my heart from beating so fast again — faith so that I could just … *trust.* I mean, I had three healthy babies already. Why shouldn't I expect and anticipate great news? Most likely, all is well, and I should enjoy being able to see the person growing inside me — reminded that our great God is the one who knits us together in the womb. So, I prayed, almost begged God, that my baby would be healthy, with nothing missing and nothing extra. Just a healthy, growing child.

I got the children ready for the appointment also, making them look as presentable as possible, with clean shirts and clean faces without traces of their last meal. As quickly as Ben walked in the door from work, we walked right back out in hopes of making it on time.

I didn't want the kids coming in for the ultrasound. I wanted it to be just Ben and me. *In case* there was anything wrong, I didn't want them to be in there. I don't know why — maybe to protect them. My grandmother was going to meet us there to help with the kids. But as we talked on the way, we decided the kids would love to get a peek at the baby. I decided in my spirit to be OK with it, to go with it and let myself trust God — and *enjoy* it.

After checking in at the main desk and getting called back, I was eventually on the table as the sonographer put warm gel on my lower abdomen. Would she be talkative, or one of the ones who doesn't say much and leaves much guessing to the patient? I hoped she would be warm and give us honest details of what she was seeing.

It's so hard to lie there and not know what they are seeing — you know, when they don't say anything and just stare at the screen. It's terribly awkward and nerve-wracking. Tell me the details! I don't want to wait to hear from the doctor. Tell me what you see!

I could feel my stomach doing flips. The first peek at the baby. I was praying that his or her developing anatomy would be measuring correctly and that nothing would be missing.

"I think it's a boy!" said one of the children.

"I think it's a girl!" said another. Lots of chatter and excitement from my little loves filled the room.

The kids, not shy at all, quickly told the sonographer all their thoughts. They were just so excited, so cute, and so thrilled to be a part of it.

"Well, we usually do this at the end," she said with enthusiasm, "but why don't we just find out right now? I want to know too."

She had pretty blonde hair and a smile on her face. She seemed like she was enjoying this just as much as we were.

Oh, I liked her. She was real. I knew from that point that I could calm down. She would be real with us. I could tell.

I felt my fears melt away — I allowed myself to smile and have fun. Everyone else was, I needed to as well.

"Well…" she said, pushing the wand around my stomach, back and forth, and pausing to get a good view. We could suddenly see a baby on the screen. A baby … my baby. I lay there seeing all four of my children in front of me. Goodness, I am blessed!

"It looks like you have a little girl!" she said excitedly.

Jumping up and down was my little Arianna. Bouncing and bouncing around the room, my daughter was full of joy for that sister she so badly wanted and believed she would receive.

"I am shocked," I say with tears flowing from my eyes. "I can't believe it! I really thought it was a boy!"

I was beyond excited to know who was in me. I was so thrilled. I was so happy to see my children jumping and talking. Ben, all smiles. A little girl. Another little girl. *Oh*, I thought to myself, *I love my boys and all they bring. And I love my girl too. Another one will be just so fun.* Thank you, God. Thank you for another gift. Thank you for this precious, precious gift you have given me.

The sonographer proceeded with the rest of the ultrasound, measuring all the little baby parts and saying they were *beautiful* and *perfect*. Exactly what every mother wants to hear. From what she could tell, and from our interpretation of all she had to say, things looked perfect.

I, again, started to sweat, my heart pounding from all the excitement and good news. I wanted to jump up and down. A healthy baby girl.

We sat in the waiting room to wait for the doctor, and I just had to send out text messages to share the news. All the responses were of excitement and joy. Oh, how fun! A new life. A new little lady for our family.

The doctor came in after a bit and confirmed our news. It was a healthy baby girl, with a due date that matched the one given at our previous ultrasound.

"So you wanted to have a VBAC?" he asked me as he looked over the notes in my chart on his tablet. He looked confused and troubled — he was the one who told me I couldn't have one. But *why* are we discussing this?

"Yes, but you said I wouldn't be able to do that here." I was surprised he would even bring it up. Why are we going over this again? It was so weird — we had already covered this topic. It really caught me off guard.

"Yes, I'm not sure why that's in your notes. There are too many risks involved with that — you would need to have another c-section. I'll just take this out of here." He continued correcting the chart.

I looked at Ben and said nothing. He was looking at me wondering what was going on, if I knew something he did not.

I was silent. As much as I respected this doctor and admired him, I was so taken aback that he mentioned *nothing* about the risks of repeat sections. Nothing at all.

We went over everything, and the doctor again confirmed the baby looked great, the due date was correct, and he congratulated us again.

"Well, we will see you again in four weeks."

"OK, thanks," I told him, not knowing how to respond.

I felt awkward — almost guilty — as I knew I would not be coming back. It was a strange feeling since this doctor and his office were indeed wonderful. They helped bring my babies into the world. But I had to remember that it was a business, and, really, we had no other ties than choosing (or not) to pay them for my care.

Lacking the confidence and the emotional strength to tell my doctor in person about my future plans, I decided later to write a letter thanking him and explaining my choice for the rest of the care for my pregnancy. I would tell him how great he was to me during my prior pregnancies, which he was. How much I appreciated him, which I did. But for reasons in my own heart, I needed to pursue a VBAC.

Dr. Marks would be writing a letter as well, and I felt it only right and respectful to write one myself. I just couldn't bear to say anything in person and allow myself to be vulnerable in such a delicate situation. I didn't want the words of others to pierce my heart in a discouraging way. I wanted to protect myself and my emotions. I knew that this journey would change my life, and I only wanted those on board to speak truth to me about it.

I walked out of that office, through the door, leaving behind the "safety" of a scheduled cesarean and toward the unknown journey of a VBAC. I had no one to guide me. No one to hold my hand, to tell me it would be all right. I chose to walk this road alone, trusting in God. I knew my husband had my back, but no one would experience the thoughts, emotions, fear, self-doubt, joy, anticipation, worry, and more that I would face. And no one would be there to tell me it was OK.

It was my road to walk alone. Thankfully, I had the best guide. My Heavenly Father, who promised to never leave me nor forsake me. He had been faithful to me through each trial and struggle in my life. Through each decision and every minute detail, He would be the one to comfort me and tell me what to do. He would be the one I would approach with my questions, my fears, my hurt, my uncertainties. He was the one who would slow and steady my heart. He would be the one to keep me strong when I felt weak. In Him I was safe and secure. And I truly could rest in that.

Eleven

As soon as Dr. Marks was on board, I called Katie, the doula, and secured her for the birth. What a miracle: I had found a doctor and a doula in the same day.

I felt over-the-top excited and was really ready to prepare for the birth. Preparation tends to give me a sense of security. I thought that if I did something positive in getting ready for my "labor day," I would have a better shot at having my baby the way I desired.

That is not to say that in order to have a safe, healthy delivery you MUST prepare. I know of women who did nothing and everything turned out. But this birth was going to change my life one way or another. A lot rested on the outcome for me — either a fourth surgery (still a possibility) or my first vaginal birth. I couldn't imagine shutting the door to more children in our family, but if a fourth cesarean happened, I believed this baby would be my last.

My protocol began with a few things that I believe really helped me. Many studies suggest labor can be made easier if mom works out and exercises during pregnancy. Every day, whether I felt like I had time or not, I would spend about 25 minutes working out. And I loved it. I really did. (I know, I can hear the sighs now). But seriously. I felt like I was doing something to positively influence the ease of labor down the road and make an impact on a successful VBAC. And I sure didn't mind the surge of endorphins afterward. I felt better about myself, and it was a great way to relieve stress and anxiety. I looked forward to this time of sweating and testing my endurance even if I had my kids as workout partners. I made exercise a priority.

I have heard some describe labor as a marathon. It takes stamina and patience. So, I decided I would train and eat like I was preparing for a true marathon. I ate according to my personal health convictions — mostly raw vegan foods and protein supplements, green smoothies and juices, red raspberry leaf and herbal teas, and lots of plain, pure water.

Again, this probably seems dull to some (or most!). Aren't all pregnant mamas eating chocolate, french fries, pickles … whatever their little hearts desire? Well, in the beginning, during morning sickness, I ate what I could get down. A steak at 10 p.m. from a nearby restaurant gave my friends and family much to tease me about since I hadn't been eating meat the few years prior. So, yes, whatever I could get down I would. I didn't eat junk, but I did stray from my typical diet. And as soon as I could, I went back to eating pretty clean. I figured elite athletes eat specific to their sport, and I would too. I wasn't here to satisfy cravings. And oh, there's nothing wrong if you do. But I wanted — I really wanted — my VBAC. I was in training for it.

I took very seriously the health of my baby and the strength of my body. I wanted no reason to have to receive even the suggestion of a c-section based on my health or hers. So, you would normally find me downing a green smoothie, some barley grass juice, or a bunch of avocados. Yes — the good fats, friends. I had no fear of them.

It just happened that my local ICAN group was having a special symposium in the weeks following my initial consult with Dr. Marks, so I attended. I don't think there were any coincidences about it. Jen Kamel from VBACFacts.com was speaking, along with Roanna Rosewood, who authored *Cut, Stapled and Mended.*

Sipping on my smoothie as I watched slide after slide from VBACFacts, I fell in love with the information that was seeping out of the words on the screen. Yes, *in love.* Overwhelmed by all I was hearing, I wanted more.

I came in knowing the birth I wanted. But as I sat there and really listened, I became angry. Angry that truth and facts hadn't been presented to me in the past at my prenatal appointments. Angry that it seemed like doctors weren't following some of ACOG's recommendations, but instead following their own personal agendas. Angry because it felt like the mother's health wasn't the top priority according to most doctors and hospitals. They had other agendas. And I wasn't aware of them before.

I walked into the conference knowing in my heart just why I wanted the birth that I did. I left there with facts in my head to back up what my heart knew. With greater confidence, I sat there knowing I was not alone. I saw many women there taking notes, just like me. Many women who were expecting and wanting a different birth than they had experienced in the past. I wasn't the only person in the world who was going against what so many had advised. In those few hours, I grew stronger, my convictions grew deeper, my confidence became a great force within me — I knew I could do what my heart was leading me to do.

While sitting there listening to Jen Kamel talk, I learned and came to understand that many doctors take their own personal factors into account when considering whether or not they will support a mother in a trial of labor. It truly is a personal decision, and who can blame them? There's malpractice insurance claims and fear of litigation, whether they even believe VBAC to be a safe option, whether or not there has been a recent rupture or lawsuit, even pressure from other hospital OBs.

I came to understand that ACOG actually recommends that if a doctor will not allow a VBAC for a patient and she desires it, he/she is to refer her to someone else who might (ACOG Practice Bulletin #115).

I also took note that "The National Institute of Health has emerging evidence of serious harms relating to multiple c-sections" (ACOG Practice Bulletin #115, 2010). Yet again, interesting! Especially since I had never heard this before talking to Dr. Sheffield. My friends who were experiencing many c-sections like me never mentioned the risks. But the facts are very clear, and real risks are involved. I was happy to know this and even more firm in my convictions.

I'm sure you could have heard a pin drop when Roanna Rosewood spoke. It was dead silent as her words and her passion challenged all of us to face our fears about birth. To write down exactly what we were afraid of happening, and to then find a partner to share it with — and then share again with the larger group.

We sat there quietly, jotting down our thoughts. I must admit, it was hard to really look deep into myself and acknowledge my very real fears and anxieties. I eventually shared my thoughts with another pregnant mom, Katie, who was expecting in the next four weeks. The two of us, strangers, sat together discussing our deepest fears, and even committed to praying for one another as we both would be attempting birth in a new and different way.

As the groups broke apart and volunteers openly shared, tears ran down many faces as women became vulnerable and expressed their lack of confidence. We could all relate. Somehow, on that day, our group bonded. Though we will never be in the same room at the same time again, it was a moment in time not easily forgotten. We faced our deepest worries, we got them out, and we decided we would be stronger than they were.

It was very moving, and very empowering, to share those things. I walked into that conference expecting some good information. I left there confident, educated, and excited, full of a passion and a boldness to keep pursuing this birth — keep visualizing it to be successful and amazing. It was life-changing for me.

That day, God opened my eyes to the beauty and awe of pregnancy and birth. On the way home, I called my friend, Laura, who had just become a doula. She truly knew my heart and desire for this birth. And it felt good. It felt good to be understood by another person, even validated for my desire — one that moved me to tears when talking about it.

God is just so crazy good. He really is. Sometimes we see that goodness, and other times we miss it. But through my pregnancy I was able to see it constantly, which is why I look back upon it in awe — His blessing and hand were over it *entirely*.

There are some seemingly little things that were important to me that God even took care of. At that point in my pregnancy, I didn't realize I shouldn't have to do anything I didn't feel comfortable with. One of them was the glucose test (which can show the presence of gestational diabetes) every woman is offered at 28 weeks. I did take the test my first pregnancy. But after Preston's food allergy issues, I drastically changed my diet and instead was able to eat a large meal (instead of drinking the glucose-test drink) before the tests for my other two pregnancies.

I told the Lord, "God, I don't know if I could ever go to another doctor. Dr. Hale has always allowed me to have a meal instead of drinking that sugar drink for the gestational diabetes test. You KNOW I don't eat sugar, yet I haven't heard of another doctor allowing this."

The Lord knew it was so important to me. It might seem small to some, but I wasn't sure how my body would handle all that sugar after *years* of consuming so little. During my initial consultation with Dr. Marks, I made sure to ask about it. His response: "First of all, I cannot make you take any tests, as you can refuse them as the patient. And as your age is only the real risk factor, and you have not had gestational diabetes during past pregnancies, I cannot see why you would need to take this test."

So, I didn't have to. Again, I felt as though the Lord knew my heart, what I wanted — even something very small and "unimportant" to many — and He answered my prayers.

Around 28 weeks, I started to see a Webster-certified chiropractor, a doctor who specializes in chiropractic during pregnancy. My goal was to feel good and hopefully get my body aligned to enable me to have a great and uneventful delivery. I have heard friends mention the blessing of chiropractic during pregnancy, and I felt it was, again, worth my time and financial commitment.

Through searching online, I found Dr. Carpenter, whose office was about a 50-minute drive from me. And it was by no accident that she was the doctor I found. Not only did she take the time to thoroughly adjust me and make sure I was in proper alignment, she herself had delivered her daughter at home. She was an incredible encouragement to me and continued to remind me that thinking positively was very important. I had no pain in my back during this pregnancy — again, a huge blessing. I know she was a vital part of my pregnancy's well-being, especially at the end, when I visited twice a week. I know God placed her in my life to help me reach my VBAC goal.

Back in December of 2013, when I had found out I was expecting our fourth baby, I had such a different perspective on prenatal care than I did with my others. I followed typical protocol — the status quo — but this time was different. For example, I didn't want to have many ultrasounds. I felt as though they were man's way to try to get more information and, sometimes, unreliable information, which can then, in turn, invoke fear in the mother's mind. All I wanted to know was that it was in the Lord's hands.

I attempted to skip out on the 10-week ultrasound, but my doctor's nurse informed me that wasn't "allowed." The purpose was to date the pregnancy (although I knew the date I conceived) and to confirm a viable one. I would have rather confirmed a viable pregnancy by doppler at 12 weeks or thereabouts, but realized I wouldn't have a choice without opposition.

Dr. Marks reminded me often that I was the patient, and that I couldn't be forced into tests or procedures offered to me. He asked to do a 28-week ultrasound to confirm the growth of the baby. But I carefully and respectfully shared my opinion about not wanting one, and he said it was no problem. It was indeed standard protocol, but I wasn't high risk, except my advanced maternal age (33!). I was able to keep my ultrasound exams to a minimum, just as I had wished.

Again, I share all of this to say: *God cares about the details.* He knows our hearts. He cares about the small things. And you can be encouraged that He hears your prayers. I am incredibly thankful for His attention to the details that were big to *me.*

I could have worried over them and stressed, but I chose to remind myself often of Matthew 6:25-26, 33:

"Therefore I tell you, do not worry about your life, what you will eat or drink; or about your body, what you will wear. Is not life more than food, and the body more than clothes? Look at the birds of the air; they do not sow or reap or store away in barns, and yet your heavenly Father feeds them. Are you not much more valuable than they? ... But seek first his kingdom and his righteousness, and all these things will be given to you as well."

Isn't that great news? When we seek HIM, when we really seek HIM, all those other things will come into place. We don't even have to spend our time or energy wondering about them. When we follow Him, love Him, love His people, it all falls into place. He changes us and in turn the things around us change.

I held on to these words even though I was tempted several times by my own thoughts — and sometimes by the words of others.

If I kept my eyes on Jesus, I would not sink. I could totally trust God. I knew I was on the path He wanted me. I would keep pursuing Him, trusting Him...

Twelve

I couldn't sleep. Again.

Ben and I slept in the main room of the apartment as our children had to share the one and only bedroom we had. We were in a time of transition and felt it would be wisest to save our money in the process of building a new home. The apartment was brand-new and beautiful. We rented from some amazing and hospitable friends, but it was, nonetheless, a lot smaller than we were used to. We made it work for the season we were in.

The window-unit air conditioner blasted us with the cold. A loud fan aided in my sleeplessness. My thoughts often ran continuously through my mind.

Life was definitely busy with three children and a house project. Life was good. But my focus, even amid that busy stage of life, was on the upcoming birth. I thought about it EVERY DAY. It was really important to me, and many times at night I just couldn't sleep. Blame it on my growing body, the moving baby inside, but my mind was moving too — and sometimes, I just couldn't get it to slow down.

I'd try to get comfortable on the couch, then eventually reach for the laptop nearby, plug in my headphones, and listen to music to settle the flood of thoughts in my head.

Maybe I made things out to be more important than they

were. But I wanted my blood pressure to be in a good range (usually it was high from anxiety) ... I wanted my baby in the proper position ... I wanted to be so fit so I could make it through labor and delivery without an epidural.

I thought about it all — I daydreamed about it all. And sometimes I would fear it. I would fear the unknown. I had never been through labor. I didn't know how to cope through the pain.

But I would still wake up in the morning and decide to work out. I would set up in the kitchen with my workout DVD going, and Ben would walk by before heading out to work.

"I'm so proud of you!" he remarked one day. "I don't know many with a belly who would be doing what you're doing."

He looked at me as I was squatting and holding on to my 15-pound weights.

"I am proud of you."

What an encouragement!

I wanted this bad. I wanted my VBAC bad. There were times I would work out and almost cry, giving it all I had, knowing the sweat and tears were for my big day. This was the best physical preparation I knew that would enable me to sustain myself through the most beautiful, awesome, and physically demanding work I would ever do in my life.

Thirteen

"So do you understand what the Group B Strep test is?" Dr. Marks asked me as I sat there for my 35-week appointment — all my children there with me coloring in their coloring books. Their three little bottoms shared the two chairs within that tiny exam room.

"Yes, I do. Yes, I will take the test."

I was trying to comply, since I hadn't with much of anything else really. Yes, we have choices to make in our healthcare and aren't forced into anything, but I surely didn't want to upset or irritate the one person who was willing to support me. No way. I just wanted to say sure, *no big deal.* Give me the test, and I will make you happy.

I now know that if he would have known my thoughts at the time, he wouldn't have said this would make *him* happy. He knew it was about me probably more than I did.

I left the office that day with no concern about my test. I felt confident — things would be fine and I had nothing to worry about.

Things were getting closer, and I was really starting to get excited. My baby girl would be arriving soon. I so longed to meet her and be with her. It had been almost four years since I had a baby. Diapers, dressing a little body, nursing again. It seemed like so long ago and, at the same time, so familiar. Like riding a bike. You just get back on and know how to do it.

I felt so thankful that I would get to be a mother again. To love another little person.

I wish I would have known more about the Group B Strep test than I did. After it was done, the results came back that I was positive for this bacteria than can live in any healthy person at any time but that can also cause problems for the baby when passing through the birth canal. The choice of treatment was to take two rounds of intravenous antibiotics during labor so that wouldn't happen.

I had a bad history with antibiotics. I had taken far too many in my life from countless sinus infections and urinary tract infections. I was also given them after each c-section. In fact, I believe it upset the balance in my digestive system and contributed to my struggle with food allergies and other issues. I did NOT want to put those meds in my body or my baby's body. However, the risks associated with Group B Strep could be fatal.

So, I decided to spend a lot of time in prayer about it. I did a lot of research and found that in the UK, women aren't even tested for Group B Strep, but rather the babies are monitored after birth. If there was suspicion, treatment would follow. From my research, there was no clear evidence that the antibiotics were effective all of the time, either.

"Are you upset about this?" Dr. Marks asked me on the phone after I had paged him with my questions. I was sure he could hear it in my voice.

"Yes," I said, looking out the window of my children's bedroom.

"I don't want to take the antibiotics at all." My stomach was hurting. I was wishing I didn't even have to think about this. I didn't want to have to deal with it, period. It felt like a roadblock after things had been going so smoothly.

He explained the risks of not taking the antibiotics and said the decision was totally up to me, but that the hospital could monitor the baby afterward and look for any warning signs. Again, he was clear to make sure I understood the risks, but conveyed that the choice was mine as the patient.

I had worked myself up thinking he would want me to take them. Or that I would be forced into something I didn't feel comfortable with.

Some friends and family expressed their concerns and tried to persuade me to treat the bacteria.

Truly, though, I decided it would not be wise to make a decision out of fear. And that is what I would have been doing. My research didn't point to antibiotics being the best answer. I would be doing it to feel "safe." In reality, I needed to listen to the Lord, trust His voice, and make my decision upon *that.*

Such challenging yet teachable moments for my heart. *Do I do what's recommended? What do most people do in this situation?* God taught me to take it to Him. Take my thoughts to Him. Take my fears to HIM. Follow Him. Trust Him, knowing He wouldn't let me down.

After much prayer, and even feelings of uncertainty at times, we believed the best course of action was to monitor the baby after birth and not use the antibiotics. Ben and I felt peace in trusting God and not jumping to treat a problem until and unless we were sure there was one.

Fourteen

"I have been having contractions for eight hours. Does this mean anything?" I texted Katie while sitting outside in the sun on the deck.

I took a lot of time-outs, at least once a day, to sit outside, soak up some vitamin D, and listen to a sermon or some encouraging music. I needed that break to get off my feet and *just be.*

"No, at 35 weeks, that's totally normal. And it could go on like that until you are in labor," she replied.

Really? I couldn't imagine enduring this kind of uncomfortable tightening for another five weeks. I responded with a kind *thank you* and said nothing else. I didn't want to appear to be Negative Nancy, but inside I was just so over it. I was exhausted from eight hours of a squeezing uterus taking my breath away. I felt like they produced "nothing" since I wasn't "in labor," even though I knew my body was doing something important, whether it was pointless to me or not.

It's amazing the way two separate bodies, baby's and mom's, work together before and during labor to bring about birth. The process still leaves me in awe and wonder — I don't know how anyone can deny a Creator exists after witnessing such awesome, real beauty as life is brought forth. Although we know so much about birth, there's so much that seems mysterious and wonderful to me.

Over the next few weeks, I was having contractions, and nights where they would last until morning ... only to stop and leave me exhausted. I felt no need to try any home remedies to speed up labor. My heart was resting. I knew my body and baby would work together at the right time.

Having countless contractions and the days ticking by, I realized this was really going to happen. There was no way out now — the baby would be coming and it was only a matter of time. I felt physically prepared. I was continuing to work out as I could. However, my regimen had changed. Taking walks with the kids whenever we were able was what I attempted, and when Ben would get home from work, I would walk an hour or more. I came to realize that while having my body ready for my marathon of labor was key, more important was getting my mind in the right place.

In the nooks and crannies of my days, I would take full advantage of my time and write down scriptures on 3 x 5 cards. The power of these words gave me strength, courage, and faith that I was doing exactly what the Lord had called me to do. Fear was my natural inclination, of course. I didn't know what natural birth would feel like, how I would handle the pain, what it would look like. But I did know one thing: God is faithful.

Of that I could be sure. He would be with me. He led me to this place. He put all the right people in my path. I had done everything I knew to do to prepare for this. The rest ... was His.

Life and death are in the power of the tongue. That was my

lesson in life at the time. And let me tell you, I decided to change the way I spoke about what was to come.

I decided that when discussing the birth, I wouldn't say *if this* or *if that* — but instead I would claim and speak as though a good natural birth was the only option, the only outcome.

"Words never lie. They live on to bless or to curse. They often return to us in blessing or in judgement. How we should realize the eternal value of words!" (*Words That Move Mountains*, Kenyon/Gossett, p. 89)

"Your words can be as poison to your own system. Your words are sometimes deadly. When you say, 'I don't believe I'll ever get over this,' you are taking poison. There is no antidote for it except to break the power of that kind of confession, begin to speak the right kind of words and make the right kind of confession ... If you think and speak failure, you will go down to that level. Your words will create an atmosphere that will injure and break you." (p. 90-91)

With my long walks in the evenings, I would take my scriptures and speak them out loud. I spoke to my body, I spoke to my situation, I spoke to my baby and encouraged her to cooperate in the process of birth. I spoke the alignment of my body. Whenever there was a quiet moment, I was speaking to my birthing situation. And I said it so much, that I started to believe it. I started to be able to see it. To breathe it. To feel it.

☙

"Have a good day," Ben told me as he reached down and

gave me a hug. I was still in bed after a long night of constant contractions. "I love you."

"Hey," I thought out loud. "What if we do go to your company picnic tomorrow?"

Wide-eyed, he just looked at me.

My due date was just two days away. We decided early on not to go to the picnic because we weren't sure if I would have had the baby yet. But, here we were — no baby. Sure, the amusement park was about two hours away, and it would be hot, but I thought maybe walking would be good for me.

"Well, we can talk about it," he replied. "I'll see if there are any other extra tickets."

"I love you," I said, and he walked out the door for the day.

I was in bed, happy but exhausted from being awake most of the night. Contractions would wake me up continuously but then would putter out by morning, leaving me tired and wondering when true labor would start.

I tried to savor the movements — the kicks, rolls, and nudges from baby. I knew it wouldn't or couldn't be forever that I would carry her. You stay pregnant for so long, you forget what it's like to NOT be pregnant. It seems as though that's what life is meant to be for you. A forever pregnant lady toddling around. And without thinking, I would sometimes take those baby-in-the-womb movements for granted. It amazed me that a few months after a baby is born, I had to think so hard about what exactly it felt like to feel a growing baby within me. Fascinating how the mind forgets so easily.

I wanted to remember this feeling. I wanted to hold it in my memory. For my body to remember these movements — the precious blessings of the childbearing years.

Her little head, I could feel, was down. Her little body, on my left side with her feet kicking my right. The perfect position for birth. She was in just the right spot, and my mind would wander and imagine what she might look like.

An ultrasound two weeks earlier showed lots of hair on her head. A little blondie like her siblings. And blue eyes like the rest, and fair skin of course. All the others looked similar yet their own. And I rested there thinking the same of her.

Still not having chosen a name, I trusted that when we saw her, we would know.

I had searched for baby names meaning *brave* and never came upon anything. I felt that word truly signified my pregnancy and that time in our lives. It would take all I had in me to do what I was about to do. To do something I was afraid of. But to trust my God, because He would see me through, He would give me the strength, His faithfulness would guide me — through the physical pain He would sustain me. In Him, I would be strong.

After our normal day of school, cooking, cleaning, and enjoying the still-summer weather, we ran out quickly to check on the progress of our under-construction home, which Ben was doing the contracting work for. It was in the process of getting framed and roofed.

What a sight to see, I'm sure: a nine-months-pregnant lady getting around a construction site. I was trying to take it all in as the kids played in the dirt — dirt that would make its way into our car, then into our apartment, and eventually into the bathtub. I tried to envision how beautiful our house would be, but I struggled to gain perspective through plywood walls.

Wow. That one really hurt. Another contraction. I had learned not to get too excited about them since they were happening so frequently. And I knew that they were only the real deal if they kept going and didn't stop. So with each contraction that came, I learned to make it through it and then ignore it.

We were soon back home with the kids bathed and in bed. No company picnic tomorrow, we decided. We would have one last hurrah as a family (before the baby came) of shopping and dinner after my 40-week check-up. Sounded fun to me. We fell asleep with the windows open, the crickets chirping and all the sounds of summer right outside.

Once I closed my eyes, I did my best to go to sleep. But for a few weeks I would often go to bed with anxiety that *this could be the night I wake up in labor*. But I knew I was ready. My heart. My mind. I was ready.

Ready to be in the moment when the time was right. Fully trusting God, I was ready to attempt this thing that I "shouldn't be allowed to do." Something others told me not to attempt. But knowing full well in my own heart it was exactly what I SHOULD do.

Ready, Lord. I am ready when the time is right. I am Yours. I am here.

I. Am. Ready.

Fifteen

I woke up and felt horrible. Like I had been hit by a bus.

I had contractions for most of the night again. Only to have them stop by the morning. I hadn't known exhaustion this way before. Maybe after having a baby, but not before. I wondered with such a lack of energy how I could endure the hard work of labor.

Ben decided to go work at the house as planned and to take the kids with him.

"You need to go walk. You will feel better. You need to move around," he had told me as I sat on the couch during a few contractions.

I didn't think he understood. I almost felt sick. Like I had the flu. And shaky. What would a man feel like in this situation? Would *he* want to take a walk or curl back up in bed? I didn't have the words to explain how I felt physically, but decided I would go for a walk anyway. I took my scriptures along to help get my mind straight and to get some exercise. I tried to tell myself it would make me feel better.

The day couldn't have been more beautiful. A small sprayer plane flew low and close to our apartment as it sprayed crops nearby. The sky was clear and the sun was beaming. It was very warm, but pleasant. I decided to walk around the lake several times on the property. I spent an hour in prayer. I spoke to my body and my baby. Speaking the true promises of God over my life. Believing and thanking Him. Trusting Him with this birth and the great plans He had for us.

"You are my strength, God," I said loudly, not caring who might hear me. "You are faithful, God. I trust You. I thank You for this VBAC. For this healthy baby."

I walked for a long, good hour and returned soaked in sweat. I felt huge — my due date was tomorrow. Lying on the floor, I did whatever stretches I was capable of. Then, beyond exhausted, I made myself get up to take a shower.

There's nothing that a good shower can't take care of. I decided I would even actually do my hair and make-up — and wear a dress! Anything to make a nine-month-pregnant momma feel better about herself. I took a long time getting ready.

Still, the family wasn't yet home, so what does a pregnant lady do in her spare time? Clean. Spick-and-span clean. And I mean *spotless*. Down to washing the comforter on the bed.

When my sweet family finally walked in the door, there was a clean mom, a clean apartment, and lunch on the table waiting for them. I made myself a green smoothie and decided to relax. I realized just how tired I was. I figured I had done all I could. It was time to surrender to the exhaustion.

After finishing lunch and my short rest, I was excited for our time together as a family. It was rare that we would go out and do things like shopping and eat out. It would be a great day.

While walking to the car, I noticed some pretty intense

contractions, but continued to ignore them. I had to stop a few times — they took my breath away. But again, I did what I knew to do. Ignore them.

About five minutes into the drive, another good, hard contraction. Shoot. I should have brought my hospital bag. Oh well, nothing I can do about it now.

"Oh no. Oh no! Something's coming out of me!" I yelled to Ben.

"What is it? What is it?"

A warm gush. I was soaked. I grabbed a fast food restaurant napkin from the console and wiped myself. Clear.

My. Water. Broke.

"My water broke … my water broke," I said to Ben. "Turn around!"

I could tell my seat was covered. There was no mistaking it. Another gush. Warm fluid.

The kids began asking what was broken and where the water was coming from. As Ben exited the highway, it all felt like an out-of-body experience. Like I wasn't fully there. Like I wasn't experiencing it and wasn't sure what to do next.

This was the day. I would be having my baby soon. I was going to meet her.

I would be experiencing labor. I didn't know what it would feel like, how I would work through it, but this was the day I'd find out. This was *my* day.

Calling my doula, Katie, seemed like the next logical step — the next right thing to do. I explained to her what had just happened, and her words came through the phone so calm and cool: "OK, well, I'll be there when you need me. Just let me know."

Her voice was happy, and steady — she was trying to keep me relaxed knowing I was about to embark on one of the biggest challenges and life-changing moments I would ever encounter. Her calm spirit was a great reminder for me to relax and enjoy this special day.

I remembered talking with her in the beginning of my journey, when I knew I would be attempting a VBAC. We had just met for the first time, and she told me what a great birth I would have. *How does she even know this will all work out?* I thought to myself.

In the beginning, this whole VBAC thing seemed so far off and out there to me. I was a woman who had c-sections. I didn't even know what birth looked like. I didn't know how to do it. I had convinced myself that my body didn't know how to do it.

But here I was in this moment. All my preparing, all my working out, all my professing and speaking a healthy, awesome labor ... it was now time to see the manifestation.

Calling friends and family on the way home produced much excitement. Excitement, questions, and advice. But I didn't have much time to talk. Soon we were home, car seat soaked. I waddled back into the apartment, clothes sticking to me, and quickly changed in disbelief. I was shaking I was so nervous, trying to figure out what I could wear to be comfortable in.

I put my wet dress into the washing machine. And as I did, it felt monumental. The washing machine I used constantly, all the time, every day. I looked at it as I threw my clothes in. It was my mom tool. One of my hired helpers. But I stood there and realized: the next time I would do laundry and use that machine, I again would be a new mom. I would be a different person. It was so weird. This very familiar machine made me realize that I would come back to my life, my job at home, my tasks, mundane as they sometimes were, and I would not be the same. This day, this event, would change me, impact me in ways in which I didn't even know yet.

I knew in my spirit that a chapter in my life was closing and a new one was beginning. And a sadness swept over me. I didn't know the new person I would be, I didn't know this new baby I'd bring home with me. All this newness would invade my life and transform me. And as I left that laundry room, it was almost as though I allowed myself to say good-bye to whatever I was leaving behind. Saying good-bye to our life as a family of five, as a mother of only c-sections. I walked out of that laundry room knowing I was walking into something new.

Lord, I'm ready and I'm willing.

From then on, it was chaos. I called my doctor's office to cancel my appointment and shared the reason why — that I would come in when I was ready. I received, and missed, a call from my doctor a few minutes later.

I paged him back, nervous about what he might say.

He asked that I call in every couple of hours to update him. And he was totally fine with me staying at home in these beginning stages of labor.

Why did I worry so much and get so nervous? I am in *good* hands. I am in *God's* hands.

I was more than happy to follow his instructions. He explained, after hearing the details, that all seemed great and normal for this point in labor. My body shook. My nerves. As the contractions came and went, and the fluid continued to gush, my body physically was showing signs of working ... and at moments I was still in disbelief. This experience seemed so foreign to me. So new. So different. Again, I felt outside of myself, trying to comprehend this was *the* moment I had worked for and trained for in all aspects. The dreaming, wishing, visualizing was bearing fruit. It was my present. It was my *now*.

Making my labor tea and attempting to finish packing my bag, I visited the bathroom often — those contractions squeezed my bladder — or so it felt. Questions from Ben, from the kids, within my own mind, racing, and my phone ringing off the hook ... I decided to go outside on the deck with my music.

Sitting there with my eyes closed, I tried to get my body to relax as the sun beat down on me. It was about 4:30 in the afternoon. The sweet neighbors we rented from came over to see how I was doing and to offer encouragement. It was very comforting to know so many people cared about and loved me. It helped me know I wasn't alone. Even though I had to do this alone, experience this in my own way, I was thankful for the affirmation and concern I had from others. It brought me much peace.

My ears listened to the same songs I had listened to in the months leading up to this much-anticipated day. The worship music that focused me, that encouraged me, streamed through my headphones right into my heart. And I just cried.

I'm scared.

I'm so scared.

Can I do this?

I doubted myself. There was no turning back, no more wondering. I didn't have to guess if I was in labor. I was. After days and nights of waiting through all those drawn-out yet fizzling contractions. This was it. And this moment, and the next few hours ahead, were what I had been waiting for, praying for. They were here … and I suddenly didn't feel quite ready anymore.

The door beside me opened, and Ben came out. The person who kept me strong. As he walked over, he asked, "Do you need more water?"

I just looked at him, wanting some encouragement.

"No, I'm good," I replied. I looked down, my eyes wet.

"I really think you need to stop taking phone calls and just rest. You need to keep your energy up."

I knew he was right, but when the important people, like your dad or sister, called to check in, you take the calls.

When you tell others a baby is on the way, people get excited. I understand that. It's fun. It's exciting knowing how mom and baby are doing. If there are any changes. If it's getting closer. If progress is being made. But I had to stay focused on resting and staying calm as my body did its work. I knew the major importance of that. I realized I needed to take that part seriously and just let myself … be.

"You should go to the hospital," one family member said. It was only about three hours after my water broke. But I knew once I got there, the interventions would await me. Being there wouldn't make me have the baby any quicker or better.

I was thankful my doctor told me to stay home as long possible, to labor there and stay away from any unnecessary interventions. And that's what I did, now on my birthing ball. But how long? How long do I stay here? When will I know to go? We did have an hour-long drive, but my contractions were definitely manageable.

"They will start to get where you can't talk through them," Katie told me over the phone when I called to check in with her. I listened to her instructions, trying to imagine what that might feel like. I was walking from room to room doing things like packing, tidying up — anything I could do to prepare. But I couldn't focus. I just kept walking. Feeling shaky and nervous. Unsure.

"Even in between the contractions you won't want to talk."

OK. I still didn't know what she meant but figured I would when I got there.

My mom came to help watch the kids. Super helpful. It was also quite the coincidence that there was a large party right outside our apartment door. A birthday party for our pastor. The kids were running in and out, slamming the door. My mom would ask questions as she was helping with them. My patience for noise, really any sound at all, was fading fast.

"Please don't talk when I am having a contraction," I said to any and every person around me.

And people kept talking. I didn't feel nauseous exactly, but I can only describe it like having the flu — feeling like you are about to be sick. Any noise or conversation would send me to the brink of throwing up. I needed the quiet to make it through the strong squeezes that kept coming along in the attempt to open up my body and bring that baby out. They didn't feel good, and I wanted outside stimulations kept to a minimum. I craved the quiet, but it was difficult to come by.

The contractions hurt to the point that I could not stand during them, so that birthing ball and I became quite good friends. The ball helped me make it through them.

"I think it's time to call Katie," I said. "I'm not sure what to do. I think I might need her."

It was 7:30 by then, about five hours after my water had broken. Yet the time had gone so fast.

As I continued to labor through each contraction, I was excited. Excited to be here at this very time. A turning point for me. And yet, there was uncertainty in my heart about the unknown. I wasn't completely aware of all that was going on around me, but I knew Ben was packing up the truck and everything was ready to go for whenever I made the call.

"What do you think?" my mom asked. She wanted to know how badly they were hurting and how soon the baby would be here.

"I have no idea."

Still able to speak in between the contractions. I tried to sip my red raspberry leaf tea and had my headphones on to drown out noise. The worship music was so good for me. It soothed me. It made me more aware of God's presence. I know that He never leaves us, that He is good, that He is faithful. But having my music kept my mind on the good and true rather than the fear.

I had to make decisions minute by minute about where I would let my heart and my mind go. Would I be afraid, or would I take one contraction at a time and trust God? My faithful Father, who had led me, blessed my pregnancy, led me to a doctor and doula, who kept me healthy and strong … I chose to trust Him. To set my mind on things above. To think of the good, true, and pure.

I heard a knock at the door — Katie had arrived. She sat next to me.

"How are you feeling?"

"I don't know. This hurts. But I have no idea when to go to the hospital. And the drive — I don't want it to be horrible." I stopped for another contraction.

"I just can't stand or move through them." I am sure I was wincing as I said those very words to her. It was getting darker in our apartment. The sun would be setting soon. The clock was ticking. For some reason, the night coupled with the unknown didn't reassure me. It bothered me to think about going to the hospital in the middle of the night. I am a homebody. I like my own home, my little apartment. The safeness. The security.

"Why don't you try putting your arms around Ben's neck as you stand next to him, and he can support you through the next contraction?" she suggested.

Still, it was hard for me to stand. It felt much better to be on my ball. I knew I was supposed to be focusing on my baby and labor, but I kept thinking of my children, outside, and what they were doing. The neighbors were watching them, but even in labor I was wondering how they were.

"You have a high pain tolerance," Ben said to me. "Maybe you are farther along than you think."

That was sweet of him to say, but I didn't feel like I was close to the end. If I were, it seemed as if the pain should be way worse.

My mom, on the other hand, was preparing a bottle of olive oil for me to use so I wouldn't tear in case I happened to deliver in the car. A part of me chuckled inside. *No, Mom. I'm not having a baby in the next few minutes, and even if I were going to, I probably wouldn't be concerned with using that olive oil.*

After a few more contractions, and more talking through it with them, I decided it was time to go. Not because of the pain, but because I couldn't handle the noise and other distractions. I *needed* the quiet. I was ready to be alone, ready to completely focus. And I didn't want to have to worry about making it to the hospital late. Plus, I knew I would need to go at some point, it might as well be now.

But could I relax at the hospital? Would I progress or move backward? And how am I going to get out to the car?...

I was a little concerned what others would think. That party going on outside, with lots of people … I'd need to pass them to get to our vehicle. That could be interesting. If I had a contraction, I would have to sit on the ball in front of everyone. Maybe in the middle of the basketball court, wincing. Now that could be awkward. There was no standing, no dancing, no swaying as some women did. I could not be graceful or beautiful in the middle of it. The best thing for me was that ball. Me on the ball — just making it through the next one.

Katie advised me to head out there as quickly as I could before the next contraction. And I did. And I ran, with the ball. If I didn't make it, I could use it.

Praise God! I made it gracefully there without needing to stop along the way. As the party guests shouted *good-bye* to me, I jumped into the passenger side of the truck. Another contraction hit.

Off we go. The squeezing in my abdomen hurt, but seemed bearable in the truck. I decided gripping the dashboard would be my best coping mechanism. And during the breaks, I made sure we were headed in the right direction, since Ben had only been to one appointment with me.

The orange sun began to set — the brilliant colors of the sky began to change. As day turned to night, moon and stars in tow, my heart felt the uncertainty of what was ahead. I felt the darkness around me, and I tried to keep my fears in check. One contraction at a time, one moment at a time. We were getting closer to the hospital … and I was not sure what to expect once we arrived.

Sixteen

"Do you want to walk or would you like a wheelchair?"

They say walking during labor is good. Any movement is good. But the wheelchair sounded good too. I couldn't answer them or make up my mind. I just looked at the nurse who asked me. I didn't have it in me to make such a simple, unimportant decision.

Being in labor, arriving at the hospital, not knowing what would come next … I wasn't even able to figure out whether I wanted someone to help me get admitted. It was such a weird feeling not being able to decide. Either by wheelchair or with my own two feet, with the contractions it wasn't going to be easy. It would hurt no matter what.

I decided on the wheelchair, but within seconds realized I wanted out. So I walked toward Labor and Delivery and used my ball when needed. I absolutely could not walk through them — I could hardly stand.

Dr. Marks knew we were coming — Ben called him on our way. As a result, we didn't have to visit Triage and instead went straight to a room.

We got settled — I put on my own pretty pink pusher gown and some fashionable non-slip hospital socks. I had learned at the ICAN Symposium in April to NOT wear the standard hospital gown. So I didn't. I wanted to be as comfortable as possible, but also wanted to be seen as *me*, not just another person in another standard gown having another baby. I wasn't a sick person who needed care and treatment. I was a mother about to birth a baby, but in a brand-new way.

I had worn the gowns before, to deliver my babies by cesarean. But not this time. No, this time was different. I would be in control this time. Not a doctor, not a nurse. Decisions this time were mine to make. I wanted that to be clear, to be known. I wanted others to know this was *my* birth.

I was very aware of my surroundings during and between contractions. A lot of women say they feel like they are somewhere else, in their own world. The air felt crisp and cool, the hospital seemed quiet with little activity in the hall. It felt very relaxed to me — not the normal hustle and bustle of daytime. Mentally this was good for me — it allowed me to feel calm and relaxed.

The room was quite large and pretty standard. No windows, which was fine, and nothing too fancy either. The bed was ready for when I'd need it. I grabbed some pads from it and put one underneath me and another on top of my birthing ball — I wanted to spend my time there, at least in the beginning. I had no idea how I would deliver the baby, position-wise. I only imagined it wouldn't be in the bed. I would be some awesome person who delivered squatting, standing up, or on all fours. Any place but the bed. That's what the hospital liked you to do, and I didn't want to go the standard route.

Music very much motivates, calms, and comforts me. Knowing this, Ben was working immediately on setting up his laptop to get my playlist going, and Katie was taking care of the lighting and making sure I was comfortable.

Back on my ball and in my zone, a male nurse came in and talked to me about drawing bloodwork, getting the heparin lock in, and so forth. He sat down in the middle of the room next to a computer and went through everything.

Great. A male nurse checking me constantly. I'm so not into this. As cheerful as he was, I really didn't want a man tending to me — no offense to the men. I had the one I needed, Ben. And I didn't even want to be checked much since I had Group B Strep. Constant cervical checks were not what I wanted, for fear of introducing the bacteria to the baby now that my water had broken.

Thankfully, once my blood was drawn and all the mandatory things were taken care of, Dr. Marks came to check on me.

"I really don't want to be checked," I said as I looked up at him from my ball. "I don't want to know my progress and get discouraged if I'm not where I want to be."

My mind went back to our conversation about my hopes and needs for this birth.

"You don't understand," I had told Dr. Marks back at my 35-week appointment. "I can't have any students observing me and any additional people. This will be a turning point in my life and will have a lot to do with my future and more children. This is really huge for me. I am sorry, but I cannot have students in there."

He probably thought I was another hormonal pregnant mother. I'm sure he sees crying, tears, and more with all the emotion running through our bodies. Or maybe he doesn't. Maybe most are compliant and put all their trust in their doctors and do what is asked of them.

But I couldn't. I just couldn't say, "No, it's OK. Students are fine." I couldn't. Too much rested on it. I had to say how I felt and not attempt to please *him* over *me* — even as thankful as I was for his help with my VBAC. At that appointment, I realized was coming to terms with my people-pleasing tendencies. This time, I had to do what was right for me.

"Don't overthink this," he told me as we sat in his office. "Your body knows exactly what to do. You just need to relax."

"Well," he said to me as I sat on my birthing ball, my eyes closed through a contraction. "We will have the anesthesiologist come in and talk with you in the event we do a c-section."

I'm sure I looked like every other pregnant woman in labor. Sitting there, concentrating through the rushes of pain inside. On the outside, I looked just like the others. Yet no one knew what I was going through. Yes, the contractions hurt. Yes, many women feel them and have felt them in order to bring and give life. Yes, this is normal. I suppose every mother goes through some sort of spiritual process. But for me, in my heart, my soul was connecting with God. In deep ways. Ways I can't even explain.

Through the physical pain, and the emotional fear I had to continually tell to leave, my soul was looking to Him. I was looking to God, looking to Jesus and His eyes to calm me and strengthen me. I knew there would be a conclusion to this labor. I knew this was it. But I was leaning on Him. I was thinking on His words to me. My heart was heavily worshipping Him for who He was and trusting Him for what He was doing in my body and in my life.

A song played in the background and brought me comfort. He left the room after our brief conversation, and I was back in my zone.

I agreed to listen and speak with the anesthesiologist — it was just part of the procedure. He came in and was so warm and kind. He, too, had a heavy accent like so many others I had come in contact with during my appointments.

Between contractions, I attempted to smile politely at him, to reciprocate the kindness. I listened to his words as he explained the possibilities of what lie ahead. I had heard a lot of it before, with the births of my other children. I knew the c-section route better than I wanted to.

After he left and I made it through another wave, I looked at Ben and Katie. "He was so nice. But I will NOT be needing him."

I said it with confidence. I said it out loud, but I said it in my mind and heart also. I had to. I had to have the words come up out of my body and into the air, back into my ears and down into my soul. I was proclaiming, I was professing, that nothing besides victory with my VBAC would be the outcome for me.

"Do you realize that multitudes of people fail in life because they speak failure? They fear failure and allow their fear to overcome their faith.

"What you say locates you. You will not — you cannot — rise above your own words. If you speak defeat, failure, anxiety, sickness, and unbelief, you will live on that level. Neither you nor anyone else, no matter how clever, will ever live above the standard of their conversation. This spiritual principle is unalterable.

"If your conversation is foolish, trifling, impractical, or disorganized, your life invariably will be the same way. With your words, you constantly paint a public picture of your inner self. Jesus said, 'out of the abundance of the heart the mouth speaketh' (Matthew 12:34)." *Words That Move Mountains*, page 111

I spoke to my mountain of labor and believed a VBAC would come to pass. It was my marathon, and there was no room for error in my speech or thought. I had only one option. I knew a VBAC was my outcome. I said it no matter what tempting thoughts of defeat, failure, or fear came to my mind. I told those thoughts *no* and spoke the words that were powerful, positive, and victorious.

Every so often Katie would take my red cup of tea and put it next to my mouth. It was hard for me to think of drinking and hydrating myself, but I knew it was important. Sitting there, in the midst of worship music, I felt best doing circles during my contractions. And I mean extreme circles. They were really starting to hurt. I tried to sing during my breaks, just quietly to myself. To worship the Lord in my heart.

Even though I was in a hospital with a lot of people who,

many would say, were experts in medicine, I knew that I was in the King's hands — and His were the best of all. I knew my baby was under His care and protection, and that was what made me feel ultimately secure.

I looked at Katie at one point in between contractions and told her, "I don't know if I can do this anymore."

Little did I know that I had a ways to go ... and if it hurt now, it would hurt more in a few hours.

I kept an eye on the clock. The hours passed as I experienced one contraction after another. One contraction down, one step closer to meeting my baby. When my other children were born, I met them as they were wrapped tightly in their blankets, all cute and swaddled. Their hats on, clean, with no evidence that they had been inside me. I met them and kissed them the best that I could.

But here I was. I was doing what I had dreamed of. Praise the Lord. This was hard work, but such a beautiful gift at the same time — the work that it takes to bring a child out of the womb and into the world. I wanted to experience that pain. I needed to experience that pain.

As someone who was told, "No, you can't do this. You shouldn't do this. You will never do this..." I needed to feel it, feel the pain that brings you to tears, to your knees, so I can ever so strongly say, "I. CAN. DO. THIS."

Eventually I added moaning and groaning to my circles on my ball. The contractions were becoming stronger. The only way I knew how to make it through them was to make some noise. I hadn't planned to groan, but it just, sort of ... came out. Automatic.

"Do you want Ben to read some scriptures to you?" Katie asked me.

"Yes, that would be so good," I said, eyes closed. I knew God's Word would bring strength to my spirit and also my body.

"God has not given us a spirit of fear but of power and love and self-control."

—2 Timothy 1:7

"Though an army besiege me, my heart will not fear; though war break out against me, even then will I be confident."

—Psalm 27:3

"Thanks be to God, who always leads us in triumph in Christ."

—2 Corinthians 2:14

"I will bless the Lord at all times;
His praise shall continually be in my mouth."

—Psalm 34:1

"Let the weak say, 'I am strong.'"

—Joel 3:10

"Death and life are in the power of the tongue,
and those who love it will eat its fruits."

—Proverbs 18:21

"I will fear no evil; for You are with me;
Your rod and Your staff, they comfort me."

—Psalm 23:4

"But I trust in your unfailing love; my heart
rejoices in your salvation.
I will sing the Lord's praise,
for he has been good to me."

—Psalm 13:5-6

"My God shall supply all your need according to His riches in glory by Christ Jesus."

—Philippians 4:19

"The Lord is the strength of my life;
Of whom shall I be afraid?"

—Psalm 27:1

"To you, O Lord, I lift up my soul.
O my God, in you I trust."
—Psalm 25:1-2

Seventeen

The only way I knew how to cope with the intense contractions was to do circles on my ball. But according to the nurse on duty, it was too much movement.

"We need to get you in a different position; we aren't able to pick up the baby's heartbeat," said gruff nurse Michelle, as she messed with the monitor on my belly.

It was hard for me to respond much. All my energy, all my focus, was an attempt to make it through the pain.

In some ways, I felt like I wasn't there. The room was dark. I was in my zone, but thinking, *No, this isn't happening*. I felt like I was going to bust. Like the pain was just going to break my body in two. When I moved, I imagined I might surely die. I can't get off this ball. I am in too much pain. I can't believe she is asking me to do this. I am not physically able to move. She has no compassion for me … can't she see my pain? Where is her grace?

"Can't you wait until my contraction stops?" I asked. Any human being, anyone who has any ounce of sympathy, would surely agree. I thought for sure she would be kind and gentle with me. Have some sort of sympathy. I was getting angry. *I am in pain. Please, please have mercy on me.*

"No, you need to get there now," she said, although it didn't seem like an emergency. There was nothing sweet in her words.

Oh my goodness. I wanted to hit her. I wanted to hurt her. I, the one who won the "Sweetest Award" in ninth grade, was so upset. "LET ME BE!" I wanted to yell.

It was so hard for me to get up. I was being pushed to the limits.

I then draped myself over the back of the bed, kneeling on my knees. Nurse Michelle kept having trouble getting the heartbeat and was saying it was dropping too low. She continued messing with the monitor.

"Is everything OK?" I asked Katie. I started to feel nervous since the nurse was making quite the deal out of the situation.

"It's fine," she replied. "She keeps picking up your heartbeat and thinking it's the baby's. The baby is fine." Katie's voice was peaceful, quiet, and calm, yet totally confident.

Oh, Doula Katie. How glad I am that you are here. You quiet my mind and put my heart at rest.

If she hadn't been there, I know I would have been tempted to let my thoughts run wild with anxiety.

Michelle continued to adjust the monitor on me. She even wanted me to keep oxygen on, but never gave any explanation about why. Which made me feel like I was being hindered, interrupted. Having her there could have easily been a major deterrent to me. If I let it be.

I understood she was doing her job, but she acted like she didn't want to be there. At all. Like I was hindering *her* — as if I was in the way.

Whatever, I don't even care. I'm going to do this. I decided to pretend she wasn't around. I mentally took her out of the situation. She could fuss around however she needed to, but I decided I would not let her be my focus.

Sweating now through the contractions. So intense. The pain was like nothing I knew how to describe, but I surely hadn't felt anything like it before.

I wanted to yell. I wanted to tell them: *If this keeps happening, I think I might die. How can a human being endure this pain? Let's get this baby out. I can't do it anymore.*

I know … I know. I read all the birthing books that say pain doesn't have to be part of birth. Maybe it doesn't. I don't really know, because my experience was that it was *painful.* It hurt. And I knew the only way out of it was to continue to be in it — move through it.

I watched the monitor from my bed, keeping an eye on the baby. My heart was beating like I was in an intense workout. And that's exactly how I felt. So I was glad for all those long walks with me huffing and puffing.

Sweat coming down my face and chest, and I wasn't even moving. I was kneeling on a bed, but my body was doing the hardest work it had ever done. How amazing that I didn't have to tell it to do this — it just knew. *My* body. The one that only knew c-sections before now.

"A VBAC wouldn't be safe for you. It's just too risky." I heard his voice in my head and saw his face. My doctor who had delivered my first three babies. Our conversation at my 16-week checkup was replayed in my mind. I was there, back in his office, sitting on that table, hearing him tell me what I wanted to do wasn't safe.

I started to feel sick to my stomach. My thoughts made me feel like throwing up.

NO, I told myself sternly, and shifted my mind from that conversation. *I will not think about that. Get out of my mind.*

You are my strength, God. I am strong. I am strong. I am strong. You are my victory.

I spoke it to myself, even in my weakness. I felt weaker than I had ever felt in my life.

But then I said it out loud, not caring what anyone thought. This is my labor, my birth, my room, my story. This is about me and my birth. I call the shots. I say who I am. I say what the outcome is. If people didn't like it, they could leave.

Perhaps it seemed harsh, but I was nearing the end of the race. Every step, every pounding on the pavement, took about every ounce within me to keep going, to not collapse. To stay there and take that next step, one contraction after another. Each one more intense than the one prior. I was getting weary — I needed encouragement. And you know? My words to myself were more encouraging than anyone else's.

"It hurts so bad," I remembered my friend Abby telling me months earlier. "But you will feel the greatest accomplishment when you do it. You will feel like you can do anything."

I held on to her words. It was painful, but *she* made it and was stronger for it.

It was so odd to feel the baby moving more and more down.

Obviously something I had never felt before. I knew the only way out of it was to go through it — let each contraction come and embrace it when it did. But I clawed my fingernails across the sheets. I didn't know how to express or manage the pain. It was becoming unbearable.

"Do you feel this?" Katie asked Ben with her hand on my lower back. "It's her bones in the pelvis opening up for the baby to move down."

I could feel Ben's hand feeling my back, and I felt it, too. Amazing that my body was doing just what it was designed to.

Wow. My body is really doing it. I am progressing. The contractions were so painful — I had never come this far before. *Can I keep doing this?*

Katie gave me a wet rag for my head. I eventually threw it on the floor — hard.

Everything hurt. I was angry that it hurt — that there was nothing I could do to relieve it.

"I want an epidural." I told her. "I cannot do this anymore." I admitted wanting the one thing I had wanted to resist all along. The epidural. I never wanted it. I was determined I would be stronger. I would be able to push past the pain. But I thought I was going to die, no exaggeration.

The whole reason I worked so hard to have a VBAC was because I didn't want another c-section. But at that moment, I envisioned them knocking me out for a cesarean and it didn't seem so bad. It might be sweet relief.

"OK," Katie said.

Then I felt Ben beside me, his voice in my ear. "You are not getting an epidural. You don't want it."

I was partly glad he said it … and partly wanted to get angry with him — he had *no* idea of the pain I was in.

"I want the doctor to come right now," I said, panicky. "Right now. Where he is? I want him to check me."

I was feeling like I couldn't handle it. Earlier in labor, I didn't want anyone around. I wanted to be left alone. But now the pain was almost scaring me, and I needed to know what was going on.

Ben left to try to find someone to get the doctor.

Michelle said he was delivering another baby, and that she could check me. Ben knew how much (little) I liked her, so told her no, we needed the doctor. (Thank you, Ben, for knowing me and my preferences!)

In my pain, Katie encouraged me to lie down and possibly try to push a little.

I'm not quite sure how I managed to do it, but with my eyes closed, I got down on my side. The next wave came over me, and when I felt like I could, I gave a little push.

"She's coming!" I screamed. Yes, *screamed*. The quiet, shy, sweet girl screamed. I couldn't control it. They say modesty goes out the door during labor. I thought only physical modesty, but in my pain, I couldn't control it … and I didn't care who heard me. I wanted help! I wanted someone to take it away and just get the baby out of me!

Was I crying wolf? I could feel the baby coming down farther, but she wasn't coming out of me yet. But I had never done this before.

I felt the bright lights come on and opened my eyes — the doctor was there, checking me.

"She's at a complete, fully dilated and ready to push," I heard him say.

Those words — so foreign to me. *Me, ready to push? I am going to help my baby leave my body and enter the world?*

This. Is. My. Time.

He sat down at my feet — it *was* time. But my cervix, my uterus, had never done this before. I couldn't believe it. I was doing it. I had gotten this far.

Still, my mind said, *Me, ready to push? I am pushing a baby out? Are you kidding me?*

The doctor told the nurses to drop the bottom half of the bed down. From the position on my back, I looked at him and said, "Thank you" — that seemed like exactly what I needed to help me the most. I was so grateful he directed them to do that for me.

"Turn that down," he said while pointing to the monitors keeping track of the two heartbeats.

"And turn that up," he remarked, pointing to the computer playing my worship music.

"Would you like a certain song to be played while she is born?" someone asked me.

I answered that I didn't care! I just wanted that baby out!

Even in the pain, I realized, once again: *Lord, thank You for a great doctor. How awesome.*

"OK, a contraction is coming," he told me. "I want you to

push for 10 counts." Katie was holding one of my legs, Ben the other.

I gave it all I had and did as I was instructed. After a few more pushes, he encouraged me to reach down and feel the baby's head.

I got so excited … *my baby's head!*

I was expecting to feel a head. The full head of a baby. I felt it, but only the size of a quarter from within the birth canal. I was a little disappointed.

"That's it?" I said.

"That's good!" they all responded.

"It looks like the baby has black hair," Katie told me.

WHAT? We don't have babies with dark hair. We have white-haired babies. I cannot believe I am pushing out a baby, for one, and now a baby with totally different hair than the rest. Who is she? I can't wait to meet her.

"Would you like a mirror to see your progress?" the doctor asked.

"Yes," I decided. I thought it would give me great encouragement and motivation to keep going. I soon realized it was more like one step forward, two steps back.

I had now come to the point of screaming while pushing. I know it's not what you're supposed to do. Not classy. *I know.* But I didn't know a way around it.

Soaked in sweat, I was yelling, "I just want her out. I just want her out. Please help get her out."

The doctor looked at me, calm as can be, and said nothing.

After the next push I started breathing hard, almost hyperventilating, my body shaking. I couldn't control myself.

"Calm down … breathe. Breathe," the doctor said.

I look over to see Ben on the couch. He's about ready to pass out — a "blood sugar crash," in his words.

I look at him as if to say, *Is this really happening?*

I am the one doing all this work, and he's the one about to pass out.

There was nothing I could do to help him, although I wished I could, so I had a student hold my other leg. I was happy to see her. I had met her before. It didn't bother me that she was with us.

"I can feel one coming," I told them. I noticed the doctor looking at the monitor, confirming, and again he coached me on what to do next.

"Well, you are almost ready to have her out," someone said to me.

"Are you serious?" I replied in disbelief.

Almost ready to have this baby out? I am almost done with this thing into which I have put my entire heart, soul, body, and mind? It's coming to the finish line? I am actually about to give birth? After all those who said I couldn't? That it wouldn't be possible? That it wouldn't be safe for me? That I hadn't done it before, so my chances were low? Those who wouldn't even talk to me because it was too dangerous?

All the hours spent preparing … driving to appointments … all of it was becoming … ***worth it***.

And yes. Her hair. It was dark. All my other children blonde. All of them birthed by the hands of surgeons.

Her. The complete opposite. Like her birth. Dark hair and birthed only by my body, without help from others.

When I had imagined the birth, I would conjure up feelings of joy and love and anticipation. But all I wanted was to *get her out*. That's it. Nothing romantic or whimsical. *Just get her out.*

And then I felt her head come out, and then her body, following so easily.

"OK," said Dr. Marks. "Do you want to reach down and grab her?"

And I did. His hands helped guide her little frame into mine, and I laid her on my chest. I looked at her all slimy and wet, and I put my hand on her little wet head as she lay face down on me. Her head was so small it fit right in my hand.

Baby and mom. Her and me. Those first few moments just as it should be. *Just us.*

She was born in the early morning, on her due date, almost 14 hours after my water broke.

I thought the tears would be flowing and I would be blown away by the moment. But I was sweaty and tired. And *glad* to be on the other side. Glad to have the pain gone. Glad to have her with me. Glad to be able to physically see the outcome.

At the time, I didn't realize how completely different this birth was from the others. I had no pain medication whatsoever but was fully aware about what was happening around me. I could take it all in. And she didn't have drugs running through her veins either.

As I held her tiny body, I was in a state of disbelief, relief, and exhaustion all at the same time.

My stitches were hurting, so I tried not to focus on the pain there, but we finally had complete skin-to-skin contact. The male nurse listened to her heartbeat, and everything else was on hold. I got to be with her — there was no rush to do anything else. This was such a wonderful experience, to be in that moment and have this great gift.

Eventually she started to look for the breast. With my older children, I would see them an hour or so after delivery and immediately helped them to latch on for their first feed. With her right next to the source, I allowed her to root around. She crawled around until she found her way and started to suck. Ben, Katie, the nurse, and I sat there and watched her. It was truly amazing. I don't know how there's any other explanation of the splendor of creation other than coming from an awesome Creator — I witnessed the beauty of birth and the natural instinct given to babies to nurse.

I was able to hold her for an hour and a half before anyone weighed her and took her measurements. It was pure joy — joy I will treasure for years to come.

Soon, I found that it was just Ben and me in the room. I'm not sure when everyone else left — I was just so caught up in our new daughter.

I had endured a great time of testing — both my faith and my body. Now, I sat and watched the clock turn to 6:30 a.m. It was a new day. The sun would be coming up again. God fulfilled His promises to me. He was faithful to me and led me where He wanted me to go. And I followed Him. I listened to Him.

While I was afraid and unsure about the unknown, I came out on the other side. As night turned to day, a new baby came earthside ... and a new me was born as well.

New life. New baby. New me.

I did it. I pushed her out without an epidural. My stomach wasn't cut open. I did not rupture. I did what they said I could not do. I did it by the strength of God and His faithfulness and love. He did a miracle in my life.

Praise be to you, Lord,
the God of our father Israel,
from everlasting to everlasting.
Yours, Lord, is the greatness and the power
and the glory and the majesty and the splendor,
for everything in heaven and earth is yours.
Yours, Lord, is the kingdom;
you are exalted as head over all.
Wealth and honor come from you;
you are the ruler of all things.
In your hands are strength and power
to exalt and give strength to all.
Now, our God, we give you thanks
and praise your glorious name.

—I Chronicles 29:10-13

Eighteen

It was the sweetest moment of my life when the children came to meet their new sister.

Six hours old and no newborn bath yet. So fresh, so new, with wavy hair underneath the newborn hat. It seemed so surreal. I was tired and realized I hadn't slept since Thursday night … and probably wouldn't be getting sleep anytime soon. Who can sleep with that rush of adrenaline?

One by one, each of my babies came to sit on the bed, surrounding their swaddled sister. Touching her face, smiling, breathing her in and smelling her newborn smell. This was the baby they had prayed for, asked about, and loved even before they met her. This was the baby I prayed for. The one I dreamt of making our family feel complete.

We had had so many conversations about this little one before she was even here. Talk of our new family member had been constantly on our lips, and now we could feel her, see her, take her in. As we sat there, the six of us, my heart couldn't be more full and thankful for the blessing, this gift of a precious new life, entrusted to our care to raise her up and show her how much God loved her.

☙

As we rested and recovered the next few days at the hospital, we tried to figure out what we would name her — we wanted to see her first before choosing.

My sister stepped in to help while Ben left for errands. Putting her headphones in my ears, I attempted to shut my eyes and rest while she watched the baby.

My intent was to "rest" while listening to the worship music, but I ended up in tears. Soaked as the warm water from eyes fell down my face onto the pillow, I had to take it in. It was the first time I allowed myself to really process what had happened.

Anyone could assume these tears were only the result of the biological process that occurs when hormones begin to shift from pregnancy to postpartum. But this wasn't my reason. Never before had I sat down in my bed after delivery and sobbed simply because of the joy I felt.

It's like your wedding day. You imagine it and cry. But on the actual day, sometimes it's hard to realize you are actually *doing it.* Experiencing the sacredness of it all.

Until later. That's when you look back and realize the reality of it.

My heart was in awe. Full of thankfulness and gratitude to God Almighty. This great, great blessing He had given me. His promises fulfilled. I birthed a baby. I didn't have a cesarean. I actually found a doctor to assist me on my journey, who honored my wishes — and my experience was exactly what I wanted. I did what seemed impossible to me. With God's grace and help, I did it.

I knew as soon as she was born I would never be the same again. The fear I lived in most of my life I would not bow to anymore. It had lost its grip on me — knowing the Lord, knowing His goodness, knowing that He can do the impossible. I could trust Him as my good Father, as my Shepherd.

"See, Jaimie, I love you. I have proven this over and over to you. The cross was enough to show you My love. But I continually show you that you can indeed trust Me."

I knew from that moment on I was called to leave fear behind. Fear that had gripped me, kept me awake at night, and paralyzed me during critical times in my life.

That fear was behind me, and I would only look back over my shoulder to serve as a reminder of who I was.

Now I would walk brave. I would stand tall. I would be free.

Nineteen

"I just don't think she looks like a Cailyn," I said to Lyndsey as I sat there trying to get comfortable even though I was in so much pain. *Cailyn* was the name Ben and I had really been considering before she was born.

Many people say that after vaginal birth they were able to stand up, walk around, and begin normal life again. I had the same great expectation for myself — it was part of the reason I desperately desired a VBAC. After a cesarean section, it's difficult every time to walk those first steps. I always felt like a waddling penguin, trying only to slide my feet across the floor hoping not to engage the core muscles that had just been through so much trauma.

But after this delivery, walking around as if nothing happened was not possible for me. I didn't exactly tear horribly, but I did have a hematoma — a pocket of blood, like a bruise underneath the skin. It's rare, but I ended up with one. Whether or not that was the case of my pain or all vaginal deliveries are like this, I didn't know. All I knew was that I could barely sit down, and it hurt to get up and to walk.

"I do like Jocelyn and Priscilla," I said with hesitation. *Priscilla*, like Elvis Presley's daughter ... not quite sure what my sister would say about that one.

"Priscilla! I love that name! And she does look like a Jocelyn," said Lyndsey.

Good, confirmation that I didn't pick out horrible names. But I didn't think there was any way of convincing Ben about "Priscilla" when he returned to the room.

And I was exactly correct. "Priscilla?!?" was his response.

I sat on the bed as comfortably as I could, he sat in the hospital chair quickly eating his dinner that I had ordered for him before he arrived.

"No way!"

With no decision made, we decided to sleep on it since we were both exhausted. However, sleep wasn't what I experienced. My nurses and the baby's nurses continued to come around — the baby needed to be fed and burped, and then she would spit up and choke when we tried to lay her down.

With the next morning's sunshine coming through the hospital drapes, our sweet, cheerful nurse came to check in.

"Have you decided on a name?" she asked with an expectant look.

"We still have not decided. What time do we need to know by?"

"They will need to know by 9 o'clock in order for the paperwork to be completed so you can check out at 11."

And with that, we made our decision. We picked a name that had been on my list for the last 10 years. And when looking it up, we found it meant *courage* or *valor*.

"I just think this signifies the whole journey you were on,"

Ben said to me as we finished talking. "It took a lot for you to do this. I think this is her name."

And I agreed.

Bryleigh.

I don't think any other name could explain more than that how she came about and who she would become.

Once we finished checking out, we were on our way home, to start our new lives with a fourth child … and the first time I left the hospital after a birth without needing to recover from surgery.

As I sat in the car, I watched the hospital fade from my view out the window. The chapter on that journey was complete and closed. It was done.

Twenty

I had done my homework and had fiercely prepared to have my baby. And I was still in tears over the whole idea even after we were back in our tiny apartment.

Maybe it *was* the postpartum hormonal changes, but, either way, tears ran down my face often in much gratitude about what had just occurred in my life.

I had to "go against the grain," as they say. I had to do exactly what many friends, family, and doctors didn't think I should attempt. I went against many loving words of advice and caution, which, I trust, came from a good place of common sense, but not necessarily an educated one, nor from God.

The journey changed the absolute core of who I was. I went from a timid, obedient person to one who *knew* where she was going and wasn't afraid to say it.

I made known to my doctors what I wanted, and knew the facts to boot. I became vocal — one who wasn't afraid to say what I thought to be right. I, the shy girl, the girl who was always afraid of new things … I became brave.

I learned to not care what anyone else thought. It didn't matter to me anymore what man's opinion was of me or my choices. Only my Heavenly Father's mattered. I still loved people, of course, and wanted to hear their thoughts, and to respond in compassion and kindness. But what they thought of me didn't burden me — I KNEW what *He* thought of me. That was enough.

Trusting God like I never had before taught me that I could trust Him again, no matter what.

> "But blessed is the one who trusts in the Lord, whose confidence is in him. They will be like a tree planted by the water that sends out its roots by the stream. It does not fear when heat comes; its leaves are always green. It has no worries in a year of drought and never fails to bear fruit."
>
> —Jeremiah 17:7-8

> "Let the morning bring me word of your unfailing love, for I have put my trust in you. Show me the way I should go, for to you I entrust my life."
>
> —Psalm 143:8

God did what I thought was impossible. And I shouldn't be surprised. He DOES the impossible.

Some might not understand the significance of Bryleigh's

birth. It wasn't easy on many levels, but much praise and thanks go to my Father for the ways in which He worked that only He could.

I experienced His provision — His presence.

Hebrews 13:5 says, "Never will I leave you, never will I forsake you."

He is always with us. He has always been. He won't ever leave.

But why did I experience Him in such a powerful way? I believe it was because I was seeking Him in a way that I hadn't before, or hadn't needed to.

The same power, that same anointing, is available to each of us, no matter our circumstances or situations. He doesn't play favorites. We will find Him when we seek Him with all our hearts (Jeremiah 29:13).

After experiencing such a miracle, I was reminded of the disciples and the way they would encounter one, like the feeding of the 5,000 in Matthew 14. Jesus fed a crowd that size, not counting the women and children, with only five loaves of bread and two fish. His closest followers and friends watched Him perform a miracle, and then, afterward, had to go on with their normal lives — had to do the mundane tasks we all do.

And I'd think: *How do I witness such a miracle, see the end of this journey, and then go on to wash dishes, do laundry, and attend a Sunday worship service at church without running up to others, shaking them, saying, "You don't understand what just happened to me!"?*

They most likely wouldn't understand even if I reacted that way. I had gotten to experience something supernatural, and I wasn't quite sure about how to go on living in the natural.

It was extremely hard for me, in fact, and something I struggled with for months. I was unable to think about Bryleigh's birth without welling up with tears thinking about the goodness of God, His greatness, and what He had done for me.

With all my emotions and hormones changing, and it taking me a good three months to feel like I could walk without pain and stand longer than a half-hour, I processed what God had done in my life — done in me — day by day.

I decided I would love Him, serve Him, and love my family and reach out to others to encourage them on their own paths, whatever they may be.

God is faithful. He does what He says He will do. He does not change, but remains the same. We can take Him at His Word.

It felt so good to get my eyes off myself and look around to what others' needs might be. There are so many hurting in this world. If we all just took a little time for someone else, we could each make a big difference.

I write this to give glory to God. To encourage you in your walk, and maybe something seemingly impossible in your life. Whatever journey you are facing, God is ever so faithful and present and loving. Run to Him. Spend time in His Word and in worship. Really read it and see for yourself what it says. Don't depend on man's traditions to translate the red letters for you. Ask God to help you understand. He will. He is absolutely faithful and trustworthy.

If you remember anything from this story, I pray it's this: I am not special. God will work in your life just as He has mine. Do you know Him? Have you given your life to Him? He is ready and willing to come and work in your story, your situations, as He has mine. Ask Him. He will never let you down. And your life will change for now and eternity.

ABOUT THE AUTHOR

Jaimie Schrock

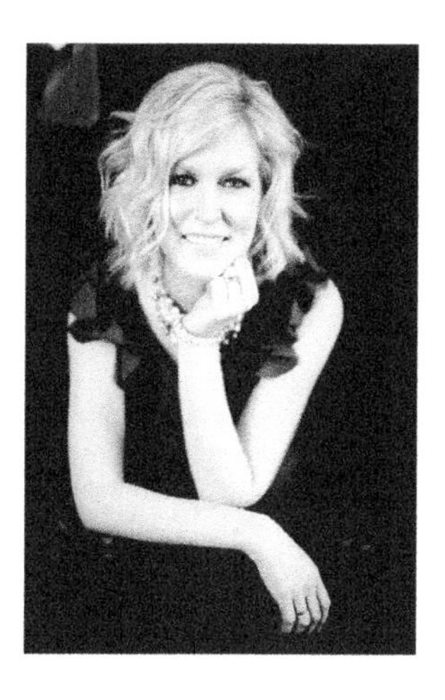

Jaimie Schrock is the proud wife to Ben and a homeschooling mom to their four children. In her spare time, she enjoys preparing meals for her family, gardening, reading, and working out. Jaimie is also a birth and bereavement doula and passionate about supporting women during pregnancy and childbirth as a birth advocate.

Connect with her via JaimieSchrock.com or on Facebook by following A VBAC Mom and Her Journey.

Made in the USA
Monee, IL
25 February 2022